Aspects of Food Production, Consumption and Energy Values

World Review of Nutrition and Dietetics

Vol. 61

KARGER

Basel · München · Paris · London · New York · New Delhi · Bangkok · Singapore · Tokyo · Sydney

Aspects of Food Production, Consumption and Energy Values

Volume Editor
Geoffrey H. Bourne
St. Georges University School of Medicine, Grenada, West Indies

23 figures and 54 tables, 1990

KARGER

Basel · München · Paris · London · New York · New Delhi · Bangkok · Singapore · Tokyo · Sydney

World Review of Nutrition and Dietetics

Library of Congress Cataloging-in-Publication Data
Aspects of food production, consumption, and energy values /
volume editor, Geoffrey H. Bourne.
(World review of nutrition and dietetics; vol. 61)
Includes bibliographical references.
1. Food supply. 2. Nutrition. 3. Food consumption. 4. Agriculture.
I. Bourne, Geoffrey H. (Geoffrey Howard), 1909–1988 II. Series.
ISBN 3-8055-4993-8

Bibliographic Indices
This publication is listed in bibliographic services, including Current Contents® and Index Medicus.

Drug Dosage

The authors and the publisher have exerted every effort to ensure that drug selection and dosage set forth in this text are in accord with current recommendations and practice at the time of publication. However, in view of ongoing research, changes in government regulations, and the constant flow of information relating to drug therapy and drug reactions, the reader is urged to check the package insert for each drug for any change in indications and dosage and for added warnings and precautions. This is particularly important when the recommended agent is a new and/or infrequently employed drug.

Printed in Switzerland by Thür AG Offsetdruck, Pratteln
ISBN 3-8055-4993-8

Contents

Bourne GH (ed): Aspects of Food Production, Consumption and Energy Values.
World Rev Nutr Diet. Basel, Karger, 1990, vol 61, pp 1–40

Patterns of Food Production and Consumption in the ASEAN Region

Geok Lin Khor[a], *E Siong Tee*[b], *Mirnalini Kandiah*[b]

[a]Department of Human Development Studies, University Pertanian Malaysia, Serdang, Selangor; [b]Division of Human Nutrition, Institute for Medical Research, Serdang, Selangor, Malaysia

Contents

Introduction

The Association of Southeast Asian Nations (ASEAN) consists of the peninsular and the archipelago parts of Southeast Asia. Established on August 8, 1967, ASEAN originally comprised of Indonesia, Malaysia, the Philippines, Singapore and Thailand; Brunei Darussalam became the sixth member in 1984. ASEAN occupies a total land area of 340 million hectares, and in 1984 had a population of 280 million (table 1), which represents a great diversity of races, religions, languages and cultures. As a group, ASEAN aims for the promotion of regional collaboration in the economic, social, cultural and technical fields. In the first few years of its existence, progress was limited to laying down the framework for the member countries to work out their concensus through periodic consultation. However, since the communist takeovers in Vietnam and Cambodia (Kampuchea) in 1975, ASEAN has been transformed into a vital political grouping that has gained international recognition. The ASEAN region is located strategically, providing important ports for transoceanic routes between the Indian subcontinent and the China mainland, as well as providing key transit points for intercontinental air routes between Europe and Australia. These locational advantages have contributed much to the development of international trade of ASEAN, which has an impact especially in the global commodity markets. The ASEAN region is the world's largest producer and exporter of natural rubber, palm oil, tropical hardwood, pepper, tin, copra and coconut oil [5].

Table 1. Total land area, population and density of the ASEAN countries in 1984 [5, 17]

	Total land area (1,000 hectares)	Total population (1,000)	Density (person/km^2)
Brunei Darussalam	527	216	38
Indonesia	181,135	159,831	83
Malaysia	32,975	15,262	46
Philippines	30,000	53,351	178
Singapore	62	2,529	4,078
Thailand	51,400	50,396	98
ASEAN (total)	296,099	281,585	

Nonetheless, a wide disparity exists among the ASEAN countries in respect of economic development. Brunei Darussalam has the highest income per capita in the region, due largely to its petroleum production, while Indonesia has the lowest. Income inequality prevails within each country, giving rise to poverty-striken segments in the population. Impairment of nutritional status, especially among young children and women, is known to be one of the notable consequences of poverty. The aim of this paper is to discuss the trends and issues related to food production and consumption with nutritional implications drawn for the ASEAN region.

Food Production

The figures on food production are depicted from the production Yearbooks published by the Food and Agriculture Organization [16, 17]. Only commodities that are considered edible are included in the computation. These include all crops and livestock products. Deductions for seed (in the case of eggs, for hatching) and for livestock and poultry feed are made for both domestically produced and imported commodities. The resulting aggregate represents disposable production for any use except as seed and feed.

Production of Major Food Staples

The production of total cereals, roots and tubers, together with the main types in each category for the ASEAN countries, is shown in table II. In 1984, ASEAN produced 10% of Asia's total cereals. The percentage is increased to approximately 15% when rice, the predominant staple food of the region, is considered. Indonesia and Thailand produced 56 and 29% respectively of ASEAN's total output, which amounted to 66.7 million metric tonnes in 1984. Indonesia has transformed itself from the world's largest rice importer into a self-sufficient producer that exported its crop in 1985 for the first time in history. The focal point of Indonesia's success has been the Rice Intensification Program, which has reaped enormous gains in yields through the provision of incentives, chemical inputs, extension services, irrigation and transport facilities, as well as by the control of prices at a level acceptable to both the farmers and consumers [42]. As for Thailand, its surplus production of rice has rendered the country to be a leading exporter, and appropriately labeled the rice granary of the world. The rest of the ASEAN countries are net importers of rice.

Table 2. Production of cereals, roots and tubers in ASEAN in 1984 (1,000 metric tonnes) [17]

	Total cereals	Rice (milled)	Maize	Roots and tubers	Cassava	Sweet potatoes
Brunei Darussalam	6	6	–	5	4	1
Indonesia	41,505	37,500	4,000	16,521	14,000	2,050
Malaysia	1,777	1,755	22	512	360	50
Philippines	11,680	8,280	3,400	3,244	1,318	1,000
Singapore	–	–	–	4	1	1
Thailand	23,728	19,200	4,150	20,349	19,985	355
ASEAN	78,696	66,741	11,572	40,635	35,668	3,457
Percent of ASEAN to Asia production	10.2	15.4	11.6	16.7	71.3	3.4

Coarse grains also make an important contribution to the total cereal production in the region. Maize is the major coarse grain cultivated, and Thailand, Indonesia and the Philippines contributed about one third each to the total of over 11.6 million metric tonnes in 1984 (table 2). In Thailand, where maize is the second major food crop, more than two thirds is exported, whereas in Indonesia and the Philippines, the bulk of the maize produced is consumed domestically. Malaysia's production of 22,000 metric tonnes in 1984 is a fraction of the 4 million tonnes produced by Thailand and Indonesia in the same year.

ASEAN's share in the market for roots and tubers in Asia amounted to 17% in 1984. Out of over 40 million metric tonnes produced, Thailand contributed half and Indonesia 40% (table 2). Cassava is the main commodity in this category, followed by sweet potatoes to a lesser extent. ASEAN is a major producer of cassava in Asia (71% in 1984) with Thailand being responsible for more than half of the total output. Thailand exports much of her cassava as chips, pellets and flour. In 1984, cassava products constituted almost one fifth of Thailand's total exports of food and live animals [4].

The livestock industry in developing countries received considerable attention during the 1970s for the following reasons [12]: (a) livestock, in particular buffalo and cattle, have the highest domestic value added; (b) the intitial promise of the Green Revolution suggested possibilities for increased supplies of grain by-products, and possible diversification of marginal lands into feed grains and fodder crops for animal feeding; (c) livestock production was encouraged to supplement rural incomes; (d) livestock products represent quality protein. However, despite extensive support, the growth of the livestock sector in ASEAN has been very slow, with the exception of poultry and swine production. In Thailand, the poultry and swine industries experienced a remarkable growth due to an expansion of livestock-related industries, whereas in Malaysia, the Philippines and Indonesia, their poultry and swine production depended on increasing imports of coarse grains and oil-seed meals. The idea of self-sufficiency in livestock products becomes illusory when the bulk of feedstuff requirements has to be imported [20], as in the case of Malaysia, where self-sufficiency in pork and poultry required approximately US $150 million of feed imports in 1985.

The growth of cattle and buffalo production has remained virtually stagnant in the region. Traditionally, these animals are raised primarily for draft power and manure with meat production as a by-product at the end of their working life. The pressure on land, which characterizes most of the ASEAN countries, works against large ruminants. Farmers' access to pastures is limited to few overgrazed communal pastures and edges of secondary forests. In Thailand, the expansion of crop cultivation into the upland areas has reduced available grazing land. Large ruminants also tend not to be favored by Philippine herdsmen because of higher risks involved in case of death or theft; also they avoid having to use common land grazing which can be fraught with government intervention [25].

In 1984, Thailand and Indonesia were the major producers of beef, buffalo and chicken meat in the region, while the Philippines led in pork production (table 3). Indonesia also was a leading producer of eggs. Malaysia's outputs of pork, poultry and eggs are at the self-sufficient level, but their production costs are about 20% higher than that in Thailand and Indonesia, owing to the price of feed having doubled between 1963 and 1983 [29]. ASEAN's production of beef and buffalo meat, and poultry amounted to 15 and 12.1% respectively of Asia's total in 1984, but its pork and egg production contributed to lower levels at 5 and 7.7% respectively.

Dairying in ASEAN remains an insignificant industry because its growth is stifled by numerous problems, such as high establishment costs, limited size of market, difficulties in establishing and maintaining productive pastures, and the need to provide efficient and hygienic transport, processing and distribution of a highly perishable product. Girardot-Berg [20] pointed out that although most Asian countries cannot engage in dairy

Table 3. Production of livestock products and total fish catch in ASEAN in 1984 [17]

	Beef and buffalo 1,000 MT	Pork 1,000 MT	Chicken 10^6 units	Hen eggs MT	Milk[a] 1,000 MT	Total fish catch 1,000 MT
Brunei Darussalam	–	–	1	2,320	–	2
Indonesia	170	93	133	220,000	153	2,259
Malaysia	14	74	55	133,800	32	679
Philippines	118	483	55	220,000	10	2,080
Singapore	–	52	14	26,138	1	25
Thailand	223	255	75	124,000	38	2,249
ASEAN	525	957	333	726,258	234	7,294
Percent of ASEAN to Asia production	15.0	5.0	12.1	7.7	0.6	–

MT = Metric tonnes.
[a] Whole, fresh cow's milk.

production as competitively as the New Zealand or Australian industries, they still choose to boost domestic production to satisfy their country's growing needs in order to save foreign exchange. The total amount of milk produced by the ASEAN countries amounted to less than 1% of Asia's production (table 3).

The littoral area of the ASEAN region is large compared to its land area. Fishing activities range from ocean fishing to aquaculture of fresh water fish and prawns. Fish, crustaceans, mollusks and other seafoods are popular among the people in the region. Indonesia, Thailand and the Philippines produced 90% of the total fish catch of ASEAN in 1984 (table 3). In Malaysia, there was a gradual decline in marine fish landings between 1980 and 1985 from 733,700 metric tonnes to 577,900, due to an overexploitation of the in-shore fishing zones coupled with the reluctance of the fishermen to engage in deep-sea fishing [41]. In Singapore, the local catch of marine fish supplies about 25% of the nation's requirement. In 1984, 25,000 metric tonnes were landed, which was an improvement from the level of about 16,000 tonnes that had remained stagnant during the 1970s.

The alternative means of obtaining fish protein is from aquaculture, although aquaculture operations are usually assessed in terms of their economic benefits and less for their nutritional effects. In the Philippines,

Table 4. Aquaculture production in ASEAN in 1983 [35]

	Indonesia	Malaysia	Philippines	Thailand
Total production (1,000 metric tonnes):				
1973	143	35	125	127
1983	199	64	441	102
Production by commodity groups, 1983 (1,000 metric tonnes):				
Crustaceans	22	–	–	15
Finfish	178	14	298	48
Mollusks	–	49	29	40
Seaweeds	–	–	132	–

culturing of milkfish (*Chanos chanos*, or known locally as *bangus*), which is favored by the poor, is very widespread. Culture of the African bream (*tilapia) (Tilapia mossambica*) is also popular, together with higher valued varieties such as sea bass. Besides these finfish, the aquaculture of seaweed and mollusks has also contributed to the increase in total aquaculture production by over 250% between 1973 and 1983 (table 4). Thailand looks to aquaculture to provide more fish and shrimp for the population. The Fifth National Economic and Social Development Plan (1982–1986) envisaged that by the end of 1986, over 500 ponds would have been established. Aquaculture production of fish, crustaceans (prawns) and mollusks (cockles) is on the increase in Malaysia, which has a vast potential from its extensive mangrove forests (for cockle farming), ex-mining pools and other freshwater bodies. An ASEAN aquaculture coordination and development project has been implemented togehter with other fisheries projects aimed at improving the stock and availability of fish in the region [9].

In terms of average annual growth rates of the major food items, Thailand and Indonesia recorded positive growth for such staples as rice, maize, cassava, pork, chicken meat and fish catch between 1980 and 1984 (table 5). Rice production expanded the fastest in Indonesia among the ASEAN countries at a 6.1% increase annually, exceeding the average for Asia during the same period (4.6%) [17]. The other ASEAN countries showed slower rates of growth for rice, with Thailand managing 2.8% per year and the Philippines at 1.5%. Malaysia registered a negative trend (minus 7.3% yearly), not only during 1980–1984, but since 1974 [41]. As a high-cost producer and in the light of the current world surplus in rice, Malaysia has been increasingly relying on imports to meet demand.

Table 5. Average annual growth rates of major food staples in ASEAN between 1980 and 1984 [5, 17]

	Rice (milled), %	Maize %	Cassava %	Pork %	Chicken meat, %	Total fish catch, %
Brunei Darussalam	0.7	–	–	–	–	–
Indonesia	6.1	5.2	1.5	1.4	12.5	5.2
Malaysia	-7.3	24.9	-17.4[a]	2.3	2.0	-2.2
Philippines	1.5	1.9	-12.5	4.4	1.3	5.9
Singapore	–	–	–	-0.9	0.2	12.6
Thailand	2.8	9.3	4.9	2.6	5.9	5.9

[a] 1980–1983.

With regards to the growth of maize production in the ASEAN region, Thailand and Indonesia, as the major producing countries, accounted for an annual growth rate of 9.3 and 5.2% respectively. These rates were higher than the average for Asia in 1980–1984 (3.8%) [17]. The Philippines managed a much smaller increase of 1.9% annually, and Malaysia's rate of output has to be considered in the light of its relatively very small production base value.

The growth rate for cassava in the region is less encouraging in that production rate declined by 17.4% per year in Malaysia and 12.5% in the Philippines, as shown in table 5. The increase rate was marginal for Indonesia and only Thailand recorded a notable yearly growth of 4.9%.

Among the livestock products, chicken production growth in Indonesia and Thailand was promising at 12.5 and 5.9% respectively between 1980 and 1984. During the same period, the highest growth rate for pork in the region was 4.4% in the Philippines (table 5). In respect of fish catch, Indonesia, the Philippines and Thailand experienced approximately the same growth of between 5 and 6% annually. Singapore's small catch increased rapidly at 12.6% per year, while in the case of Malaysia, her catch has been diminishing as mentioned previously.

Trends in Crop Production Increases

Paulino [33] reported that increases in output per hectare at an average rate of 2.9% a year accounted for 85% of production growth in Asia during 1961–1980. Expansion of area harvested averaged only 0.5% annually. In 1980–1984, a similar trend prevailed with respect to rice and

Table 6. Contribution of area and yield to production increases of rice and maize in ASEAN, 1980–1984 [17]

	Average annual growth rate, %		Contribution to production increases, %	
	area harvested	yield per hectare	area harvested	yield per hectare
Rice				
Brunei Darussalam	-8.3	4.7	[a]	100.0
Indonesia	2.0	4.5	30.8	69.2
Malaysia	-2.0	-2.0	[b]	[b]
Philippines	-2.1	3.7	[a]	100.0
Singapore	–	–	–	–
Thailand	1.6	1.0	61.5	38.5
ASEAN	-1.8	2.4	[a]	100.0
Asia	0.7	3.9	15.2	84.8
Maize				
Brunei Darussalam	–	–	–	–
Indonesia	1.7	11.0	13.4	86.6
Malaysia	22.3	8.8	71.7	28.3
Philippines	-2.5	1.1	[a]	100.0
Singapore	–	–	–	–
Thailand	6.2	2.9	68.1	31.9
ASEAN	6.9	6.0	53.5	46.5
Asia	0.03	4.4	0.7	99.3

[a] Contribution to production increase is assigned totally to yield because of negative growth in area harvested.
[b] Neither area nor yield contributed to production increase.

maize production growth in Asia (table 6). Yield per hectare contributed to 84.8 and 99.3% of production increase for rice and maize respectively. In the case of ASEAN, the region in general relied upon crop yields for increasing the production of rice. However, the major producers, namely Thailand and Indonesia, also depended substantially on area expansion for production increases; between 1980 and 1984, area expansion provided for 61.5 and 30.8% respectively of the annual growth of their rice production. Thailand, as a major world exporter of rice, responded cautiously to the new rice varieties introduced by Asia's Green Revolution embarked in the mid-1960s. In 1979, only 9% of the rice area in Thailand had been planted with the high yielding varieties compared to 78% in the Philippines and 60% in Indonesia in 1980 [22]. Most of the rice holdings in

Thailand are less than 5 hectares and belonging to farmers with limited funds to purchase those chemical inputs that constituted the basis of the Green Revolution. The result is that production growth in Thailand has been accomplished mainly through expansion into new lands, sometimes causing destruction of the watersheds [32]. In the case of the Philippines, the pioneer of the Green Revolution, increase in rice yield has been the chief source of growth as compared to the 1950s when 80% of the increase in agricultural output was accounted for by area expansion [43].

Although the ASEAN countries have improved their rice yields over the years, they still lag behind the yields shown by other countries in Asia (table 7). Indonesia's yield of 3,866 kg/ha in 1984 was the highest for ASEAN but it was barely 60% that of Asia's best yield recorded by the Republic of Korea. Thailand's yield of 1979 kg/ha was the lowest in the ASEAN region, and it remains a matter of concern to the Thai food policy makers [32].

The production increase of maize between 1980 and 1984 was due to expansion of area harvested in Malaysia and Thailand and to improvement in the yield per hectare in Indonesia and the Philippines (table 6). Maize yields are low according to Asian standards with none of the ASEAN countries at level with the average yield for Asia (2,771 kg/ha) (table 7). Thailand achieved the highest yield in ASEAN at 2,500 kg/ha, followed by Indonesia and Malaysia at approximately 1,600 kg/ha.

Cassava, sugar cane, oil palm and coconut are the other major food crops cultivated in the ASEAN region. Between 1980 and 1984, there was a reduction in the area planted with cassava in the member countries, with the exception of Thailand, which expanded at 5.9% annually (table 8). Yield improvement for cassava has been limited to 3 and 1.5% per annum for Indonesia and Thailand respectively. In contrast, cassava yield declined at 12.9% yearly in the Philippines, whilst in Malaysia, the yield per hectare has remained stagnant. Nonetheless, cassava yield of Malaysia, at 12,000 kg/ha, was the second highest in the region, next to Thailand's yield of almost 15,000 kg/ha (table 7).

Sugar cane is an important economic food crop, especially in Thailand, the Philippines and Indonesia. Area expansion was the major contributor to production increase in these countries during 1980–1984 (table 8). Yield improvement was just as significant in improving production in Indonesia. Her sugar cane plantations were developed by the Dutch, who introduced the policy of obligating farmers to rent their land to sugar mills operating large estates [30]. This system was reversed by the govern-

Table 7. Yields (kg/ha) of some major food crops in 1984 [17]

	Rice	Maize	Cassava	Sugar cane
Indonesia	3,866	1,600	9,859	85,345
Malaysia	2,659	1,571	12,000	45,455
Philippines	2,486	999	8,000	42,336
Thailand	1,979	2,500	14,970	43,140
ASEAN (average)	2,748	1,668	11,207	54,069
China	5,271	3,846	16,139	62,001
Japan	6,414	3,000	–	64,167
Korea Republic	6,475	4,441	–	–
Asia (average)	3,268	2,771	11,988	52,871

Table 8. Contribution of area harvested and yield towards production increase of cassava, sugarcane, oil palm and coconut in ASEAN, 1980–1984 [5]

	Average annual growth rate, %		Contribution to production increases, %	
	area harvested	yield per hectare	area harvested	yield per hectare
Cassava				
Indonesia	–1.0	3.0	c	100.0
Malaysia	–17.2[a]	0	c	0
Philippines	–1.2	–12.9	d	d
Thailand	5.9	1.5	79.7	20.3
Sugar cane				
Indonesia	4.9	5.0	49.5	50.5
Philippines	3.5	1.0	77.8	22.2
Thailand	4.9	2.6	66.2	33.8
Oil palm				
Indonesia	10.9	0.4	96.5	3.5
Malaysia	7.0[a]	13.0	35.0	65.0
Thailand	47.5[b]	0.2	99.6	0.4
Coconuts				
Indonesia	3.0	–3.6	100.0	c
Philippines	0.7	–10.3	100.0	c
Thailand	6.5	7.6	46.1	53.9

[a] 1980–1983.
[b] 1981–1984.
[c] Contribution to production increase is assigned totally to yield because of negative growth in area harvested.
[d] Neither area nor yield contributed to production increase.

ment in 1975, and by 1984, smallholder cane farming had improved the yield to be approximately twice that of Thailand, Malaysia and the Philippines (table 7).

The palm oil industry is burgeoning in Malaysia, providing employment for more than 300,000 people and contributing about 10% to the country's export earnings (US$ 2,000 million in 1984) [31]. Malaysia is the world's largest producer and exporter of palm oil, accounting for 60 and 67.4% of world production and export respectively in 1984. Its production increase between 1980 and 1983 was due partly to an expansion of planted hectarage (7% increase per annum), and twice as much to yield improvement (table 8). Thailand and Indonesia relied on area expansion solely towards their production increase of oil palm. The total area under oil palm in these two countries is relatively small, amounting to under one third of that in Malaysia.

Coconut is an important food crop in the ASEAN region, with Indonesia as the leading producer, followed by the Philippines. In 1984, Indonesia produced 35.8% of the coconuts in Asia-Pacific, and the Philippines production accounted for 24.5% [35]. Together with Malaysia and Thailand, these ASEAN countries contributed to nearly 71% of the coconuts in Asia-Pacific region. As shown in table 8, coconut production increase during 1980–1984 was due to area expansion, with the exception of Thailand, which owed its increase almost equally to area expansion and yield improvement. In fact, the yield of coconuts in Thailand in 1984 far exceeded those in Indonesia and the Philippines [17].

Food Availability

The food balance sheet is a useful management tool, developed for disclosing trends in national food supply and estimating the availability of food items, which can be translated into calories and other nutrients on a per capita per day basis. Data on a country's agriculture production, food imports and exports, changes in stock, amounts used as a feed, seeds and losses due to wastage and spoilage are calculated to represent national supply. The per capita supply, representing food availability, is obtained by dividing the national supply by the total population during the same period. The main weakness of the food balance sheet is that it does not indicate the differences that may exist in the diet consumed due to socio-economic, cultural, ecological and seasonal variations. Nonetheless, com-

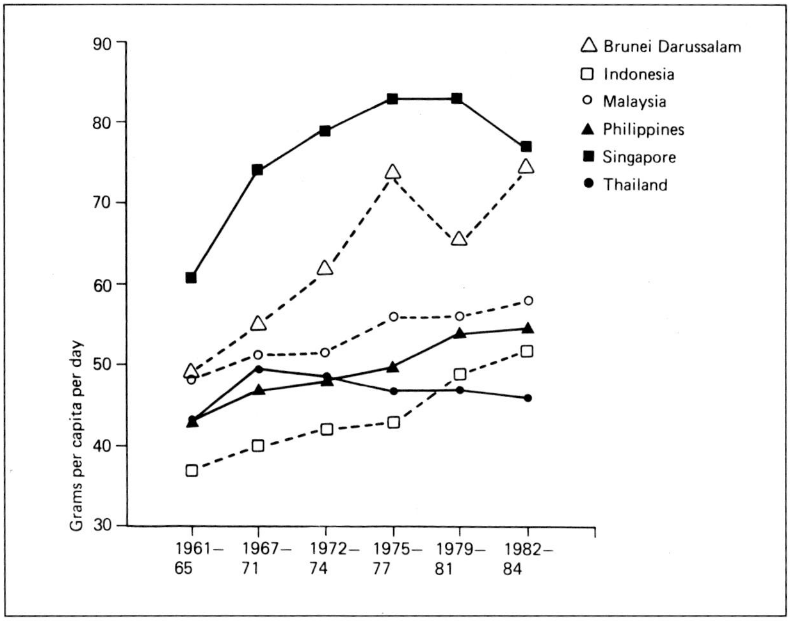

Fig. 1. Changes in availability of calories between 1961 and 1984. Plotted from data in ref. [23–15].

paring the food availability among the countries in ASEAN can provide an insight into the patterns of food supply and availability of nutrients in the region.

Available Calories Supply

During the past two decades (1961–1984), countries in ASEAN have experienced a general upward trend in the availability of total calories as illustrated in figure 1. On the average, the region recorded a 20.9% increase in calorie availability during the two decades (table 9). Brunei Darussalam, Indonesia and the Philippines produced higher increases (28–35%) than the region's average, whilst Singapore, Malaysia and Thailand showed 8.4–12.1% increases. Betweeen 1982 and 1984, calories available on a per caput per day basis ranged from 2,322 cal in Thailand to 2,783 cal in Brunei Darussalam. Although all the countries in ASEAN traditionally derive the bulk of their calories from cereals especially rice, there has been a downward trend in the contribution of cereals to the total available calories supply.

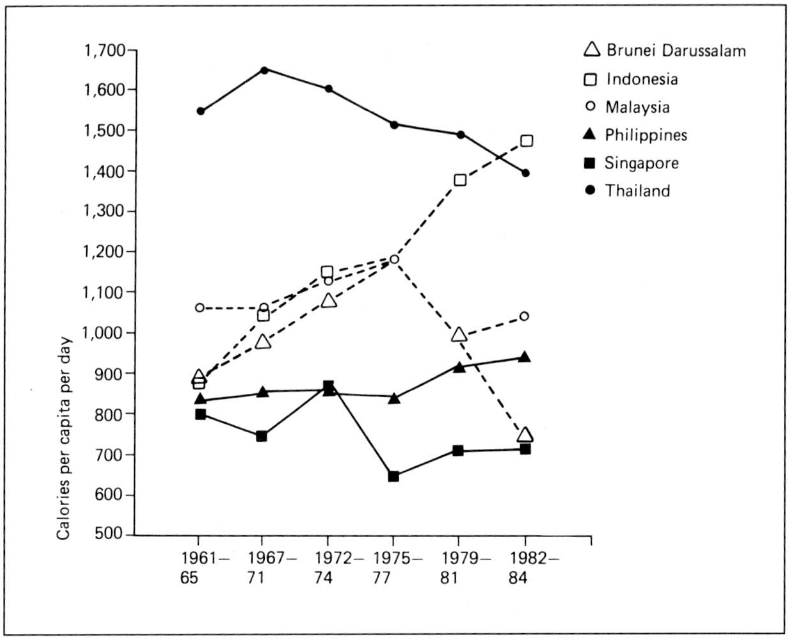

Fig. 2. Changes in available calories from rice between 1961 and 1984. Plotted from data in ref. [13–15].

Table 9. Changes in available calories supply in ASEAN [13, 15]

	Total calories available in 1982–1984 per caput per day	Change in total available calories 1961–1984 %	Animal calories ÷ total calories 1982–1984 %	Change in availability of calories from animal sources 1961–1984 %	Changes in contribution of food to calories supply 1961–1984: cereals %	roots and tubers %	sugar and honey %	oils and fats %
Brunei Darussalam	2,783	32.0	21.2	91.0	-2.9	-41.3	-21.2	8.6
Indonesia	2,433	35.0	2.4	0	12.1	-46.1	0	17.0
Malaysia	2,549	8.4	13.9	35.0	-9.9	68.8	15.4	18.2
Philippines	2,399	28.0	10.1	-5.6	-4.7	20.0	25.3	13.5
Singapore	2,725	12.1	26.2	56.0	-7.7	163.3	-18.9	26.9
Thailand	2,322	9.6	6.3	1.6	-10.3	42.1	163.8	47.1
ASEAN (average)	2,535	20.9	13.4	30.0	-3.9	34.5	27.4	21.9

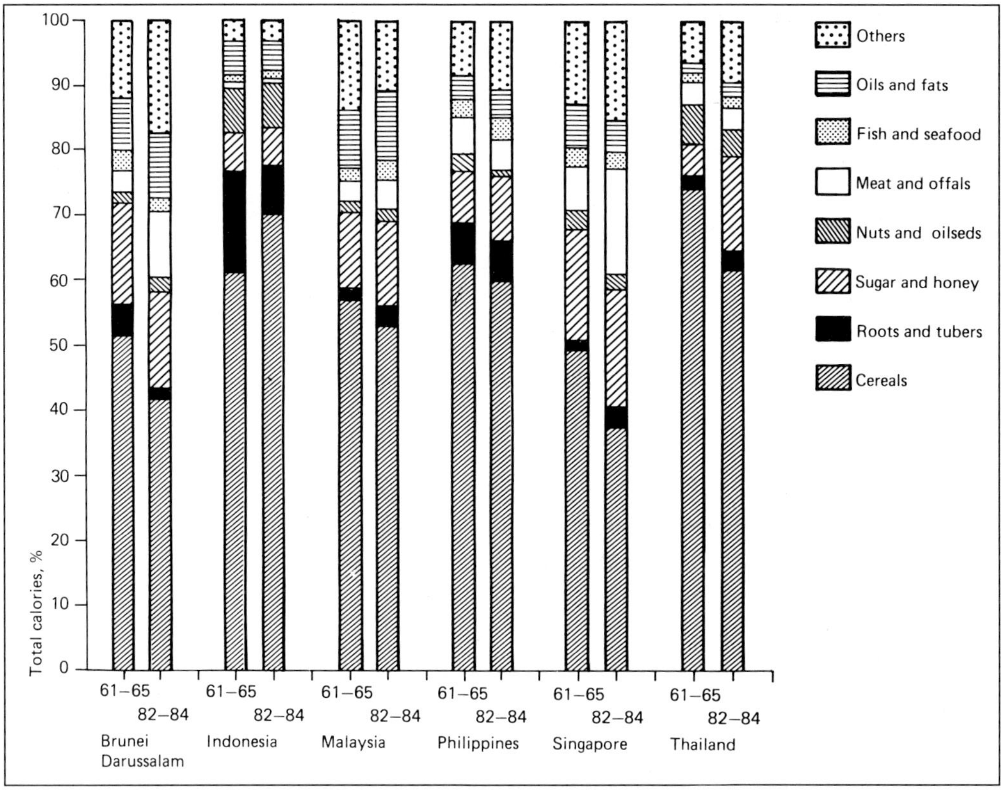

Fig. 3. Contribution by major food groups to total available calories – changes between 1961 and 1984. Plotted from data in ref. [13, 15]. Others include pulses, fruit, vegetable, eggs, milk, spices and stimulants.

Table 9 reveals that between 1961 and 1984, cereal contribution decreased in values ranging from 2.9% in Brunei Darussalam to 10.3% in Thailand. Indonesia was the only ASEAN country to have an increase of 12.1% in calories from cereals. Figure 2 compares the changes in the availability of calories from rice between 1961 and 1984, and it reiterates the position of Indonesia as the only member country to register an increase (11.7%) of calories from rice. The other countries showed decreases ranging from 4.6% for Malaysia to 15.4% for Brunei Darussalam.

Aside from cereals, roots and tubers, sugar, and oils and fats formed the other major sources of calories among the ASEAN countries (fig. 3).

Table 10. Pattern of available protein supply in ASEAN [13, 15]

	Total protein available in 1982–1984 g/capita/day	Change in total protein supply 1961–1984, %	Animal protein as % of total protein supply 1982–1984	Change in % of animal protein to total protein 1961–1984
Brunei Darussalam	74.6	51.3	52.4	9.8
Indonesia	51.7	39.8	12.8	0.6
Malaysia	58.0	20.3	43.1	14.8
Philippines	54.6	27.3	37.0	1.8
Singapore	76.6	26.0	58.1	17.5
Thailand	45.8	5.8	26.9	20.0
ASEAN (average)	60.2	28.5	38.4	10.8

Calorie contribution by the roots and tubers group, which consists of cassava mainly, increased the most in Thailand by 42.1% during the two decades (table 9). The other major producer of this crop in the region is Indonesia, but calories from its cassava supply decreased by 46.1% during the same period. Although table 9 indicates substantial increases in calories from roots and tubers in Malaysia and Singapore, the values must be considered in respect of their relatively small supply of available cassava.

Calories from sugar has been on the increase in ASEAN, with the exception of Brunei Darussalam and Singapore. Thailand registered the highest change of 163.3% between 1961 and 1984 (table 9), reflecting the country's diversification from rice to sugar production beginning in the 1970s. Table 9 also shows that contribution of calories from oils and fats increased considerably in all the ASEAN countries during the two decades.

Available Protein Supply

Total protein available in grams per capita per day in 1982–1984 differed widely among the ASEAN countries, ranging from 45.8 g in Thailand to 76.6 g in Singapore. Protein availability has been on a general upward trend since 1961, averaging 28.5% increase for the region (table 10). Thailand experienced the least change during the period (5.8%), as compared to 51.3% increase for Brunei Darussalam. Figure 4 shows the higher availability of total protein in Singapore and Brunei Darussalam than in the remaining ASEAN countries. These two countries also enjoyed a higher

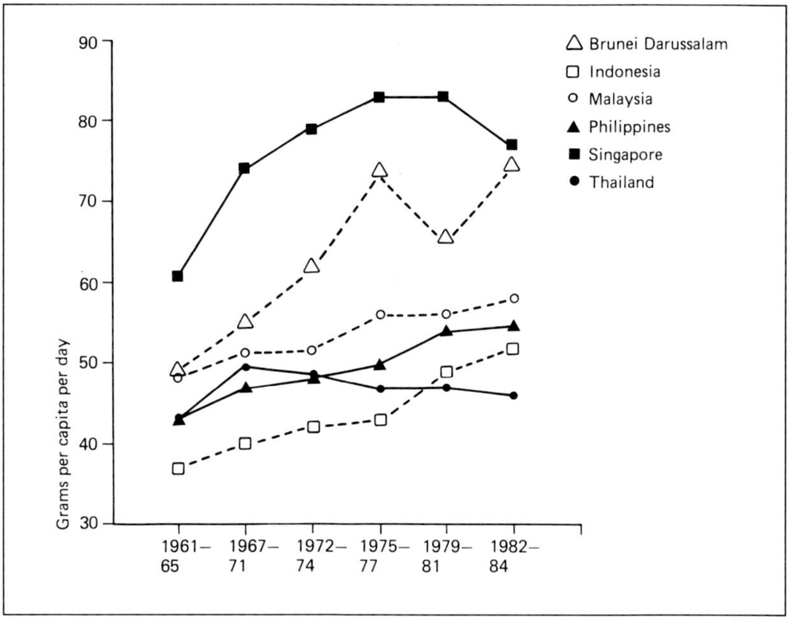

Fig. 4. Changes in availability of total protein between 1961 and 1984. Plotted from data in ref. [13–15].

percentage of protein from animal products (52.4–58.1%) than the rest of ASEAN. Although Thailand's level of animal protein was much less at 26.9%, it is significant that its percent of animal protein to total protein increased much more than the change in total protein supply over the period of 1961–1984. In contrast, Indonesia and the Philippines had virtually stagnated in their available animal protein to total protein percentage (table 10).

The pattern of per capita protein supply in many ASEAN countries during the two decades has undergone a shift towards an increased availability of animal protein especially from fish, meat, milk and eggs (table 11). Meat here includes beef, veal, buffalo meat, pork and poultry. It is mainly the latter two types of meat that are responsible for the growth of meat availability. The increased availability of eggs among the animal products is in contrast to the trend in countries like the USA [24], Canada [11] and Australia [34] where per capita egg consumption has gone down in recent years, most likely influenced by cholesterol implications. All the

Table 11. Changes in available protein supply in ASEAN [13, 15]

	Changes (%) in contribution of food groups to protein supply 1961–1984						
	cereals	pulses	nuts and oilseeds	meat and offals	eggs	fish and seafood	milk
Brunei Darussalam	-8.7	6.3	57.7	84.6	62.5	-44.9	37.3
Indonesia	9.7	-16.7	-3.5	-29.0	100.0	-1.3	166.7
Malaysia	-14.9	21.6	-84.8	36.5	24.2	54.6	56.1
Philippines	-1.2	-21.4	-52.6	-12.8	15.8	3.8	17.9
Singapore	-9.1	-41.9	-39.7	34.7	29.0	-15.1	55.9
Thailand	-8.5	-46.4	-39.2	14.7	-38.1	45.2	88.9
ASEAN	-5.5	-16.4	-27.0	21.7	32.2	7.1	70.5

Table 12. Changes in available fat supply in ASEAN [13, 15]

	Total fat available in 1982–84 g per capita per day	Change in total fat supply 1961–1984, %	Animal fat as % of total fat supply in 1982–1984	Change in ratio of animal fat to total fat 1961–1984, %	Main sources	
					animal fats	vegetable oils
Brunei Darussalam	74.9	37.2	51.8	13.9	butter	coconut oil groundnut oil
Indonesia	36.0	24.1	8.9	0.3	butter	coconut oil groundnut oil
Malaysia	56.9	38.1	36.4	-3.4	butter	palm oil coconut oil
Philippines	33.2	15.1	48.5	0.2	lard	coconut oil
Singapore	69.4	20.5	71.6	21.6	ghee butter	soybean oil maize oil
Thailand	28.2	-0.7	34.0	0.8	lard tallow	coconut oil soybean oil
ASEAN (average)	49.8	22.4	41.9	5.6		

ASEAN countries showed substantial expansion in their per capita milk supply over the past two decades. This is largely due to imports since domestic production of fluid milk has been slow to increase. It is reported that six countries in Southeast Asia, namely the Philippines, Indonesia, Thailand, Malaysia, Singapore and Burma import about a quarter of the

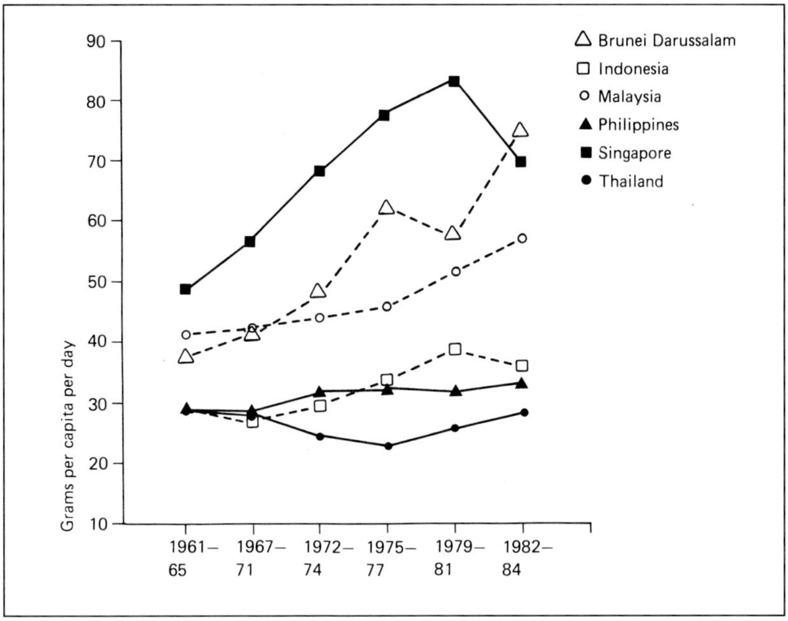

Fig. 5. Changes in availability of total fat between 1961 and 1984. Plotted from data in references [13–15].

world's trade in milk powder [20]. The same period between 1961 and 1984 saw a concomitant decline in the supply of protein from plant sources, notably cereals, pulses and nuts in almost all the ASEAN countries. This shift from less vegetable protein to more animal protein may be related to improvement in the gross national product (GNP) of the ASEAN countries. Increase in income also seems to displace fish as food for higher valued meat. Brunei Darussalam and Singapore, with the higher GNP per capita in the region, showed a substantial decline in the availability of fish between 1961 and 1984.

Available Fat Supply

Availability of total fat in gram per capita per day of the various ASEAN countries between 1961 and 1984 are represented in figure 5. Increase in fat availability during the period was substantial for Malaysia and Brunei Darussalam, and less for Indonesia, Singapore and the Philippines (table 12). Thailand showed a marginal decrease in fat availability between 1961 and 1984. In terms of the percentage of animal fat in the total fat supply, the differences among the member countries were remarkable, ranging from about one third in Malaysia and Thailand, nearly half in the Philippines and Brunei Darussalam, to two thirds in Singapore. These levels of animal fat in the diet have changed more significantly for Singapore and Brunei Darussalam than for the other members, whose levels have virtually stagnated or even declined somewhat as in Malaysia and the Philippines. Table 12 also shows that the ASEAN countries, with the exception of Malaysia and Singapore, relied on butter, lard and coconut oil as their main fat sources. These contain a higher level of saturated fat than palm oil and soybean oil which are the principal fat sources in Malaysia and Singapore respectively.

Changes in Compositon of Energy Intake

The contribution of calories from protein, fat and carbohydrates towards the total energy intake for each ASEAN country between 1961 and 1984 is represented in figure 6. In general, the percentage of calories derived from carbohydrates has remained approximately between 70 and 80% over the 20 years. In comparison, carbohydrate energy intake of Japan dropped from 72.1 to 60.3% between 1965 and 1983, with a corresponding increase in energy from fat sources from 14.8 to 24.6% [1]. Among the ASEAN countries, Singapore, Brunei Darussalam and Malaysia shared a similar trend with Japan in increasing their ratio of fat calories during the same period. The other members showed a slight decline in the proportion of energy from fat sources, which is more in keeping with the change that occurred in the USA between 1977 and 1985, when both preschool children and women were found to consume less food energy from fat and carbohydrates [24]. Changes in the level of energy from protein in the ASEAN diet ranged between 8 and 10% of the total calories. Only Singapore and Brunei Darussalam had their protein calories exceeding 10% in 1982–1984.

Differentiation between animal and plant sources of calories continue to receive interest in view of the implications of dietary fats with the development of ischemic heart disease. In this region, the average level of calories from animal products was 13.4% in 1982–1984 (table 9), one and half times higher than that for Asia [17]. Singapore, Brunei Darussalam and Malaysia had more available calories derived from animal sources than the average for ASEAN, with Singapore having the highest availability at 26.2%. These three members experienced a considerable increase in

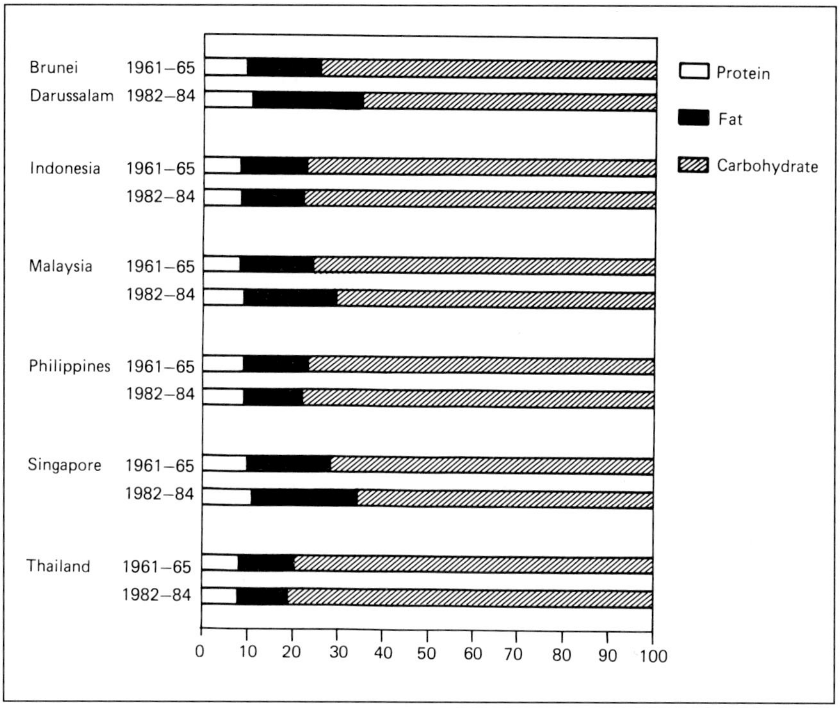

Fig. 6. Energy ratio of protein, fat and carbohydrate. Plotted from data in ref. [13, 15].

availability of animal calories (between 35.0 and 91.0%). Indonesia had the lowest ratio of animal calories to total calories and the situation has not changed for the last two decades. The Philippines showed a decrease in its percentage of calories from animal products, while Thailand's relatively low level of 6.3% of animal calories has hardly changed during the period of 1962–1984.

Availability of Other Nutrients

Besides calories and the macronutrients of protein and fat, four other nutrients have been selected on the basis of their importance in the ASEAN region. Vitamin A and iron deficiency are common in many parts of ASEAN followed by inadequate intake of thiamine and riboflavin [27] Figures 7 and 8 show the availability of these nutrients in 1980–1982.

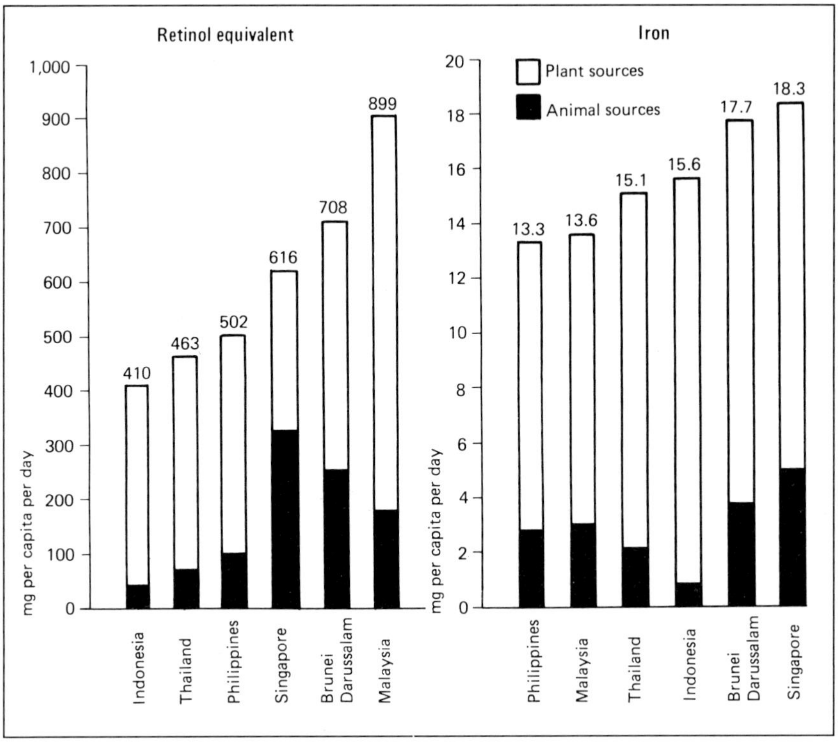

Fig. 7. Supply of total retinol equivalent and iron in 1980–1982. Plotted from data in ref. [17]. Total retinol equivalent/iron given on top of bars.

Malaysia, Brunei Darussalam and Singapore recorded over 600 to nearly 900 retinol equivalents per capita per day. They had a higher level of retinol equivalent than the other member countries because of their higher availability of animal products. Nonetheless, the percentage of retinol equivalent from plant sources exceeded that from animal products for all the ASEAN countries, with the exception of Singapore, whose total retinol equivalent was due almost equally to animal and plant sources. Table 13 indicates that Malaysia and Indonesia experienced the fastest expansion in the supply of available retinol equivalent in ASEAN between 1969 and 1982, this growth being due mostly to an increase in the availability of plant retinol equivalent. Palm oil is likely the single most important source of retinol equivalent that contributed to the substantial increase.

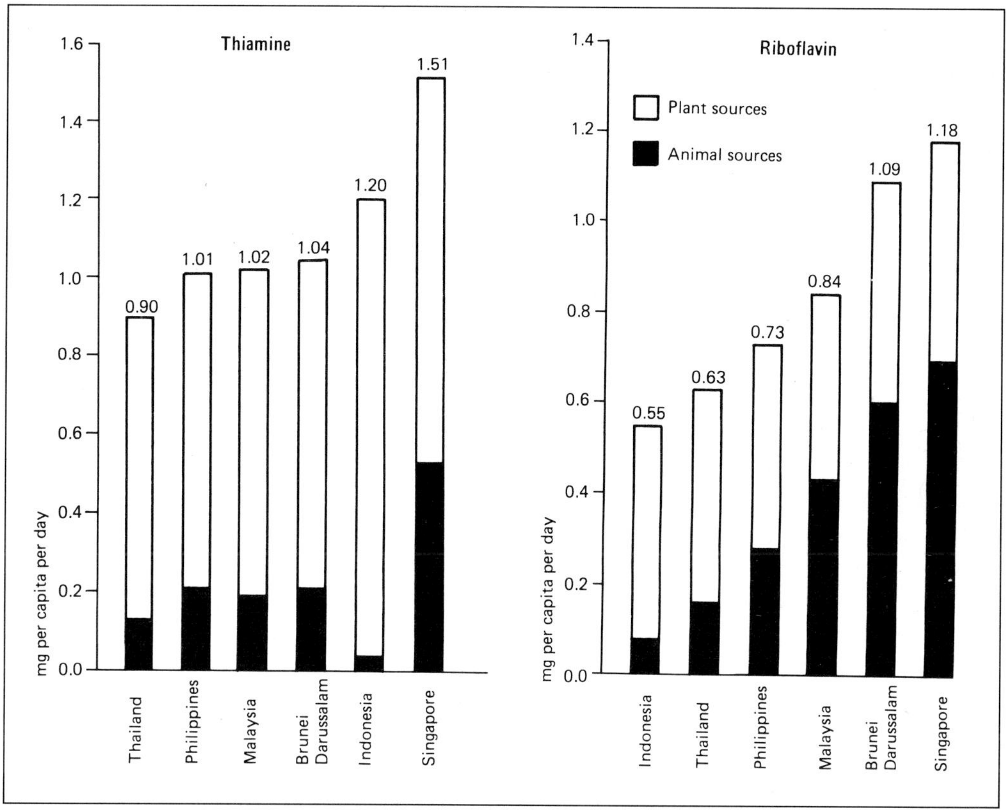

Fig. 8. Supply of thiamine and riboflavin in 1980–1982. Plotted from data in ref. [17]. Total thiamine/riboflavin given on top of bars.

The amounts of iron, thiamine and riboflavin available to the ASEAN population increased by 13.2, 17.1 and 17.1% respectively between 1969 and 1982. Table 13 shows that, on the average, ASEAN relied on plant products for 82, 75 and 58% of its iron, thiamine and riboflavin supply respectively. During the period of 1969–1982, Indonesia experienced the best overall improvement in the availability of iron, thiamine and riboflavin. Plant sources of iron in the diet of the region comprise of soybean, mungbean, spinach, squash and maize. The main source of thiamine is rice followed by soybean, mungbean and peanuts. The beans and sweet potatoes serve as important plant sources of riboflavin.

Table 13. Percent changes in the availability of retinol equivalent (RE), iron, thiamine and riboflavin in ASEAN, 1969–1982 [17]

	Retinol		Iron		Thiamine		Riboflavin	
	plant RE ÷ total RE in 1982	change in availability of total RE %	plant iron ÷ total iron in 1982	change in availability of total iron %	plant thiamine ÷ total thiamine in 1982	change in availability of total thiamine %	plant riboflavin ÷ total riboflavin in 1982	change in availability of total riboflavin %
Brunei Darussalam	64	14.9	79	5.4	80	11.8	44	11.2
Indonesia	90	73.7	96	22.8	77	26.3	76	25.0
Malaysia	80	92.9	78	3.0	80	13.3	49	25.4
Philippines	80	37.5	78	29.1	68	21.7	62	19.7
Singapore	48	19.2	74	9.6	60	26.9	42	18.0
Thailand	85	2.9	86	9.4	86	2.3	75	3.3
ASEAN (average)	75	40.2	82	13.2	75	17.1	58	17.1

Food Consumption

Data on food consumption are based on results of dietary surveys that have been undertaken over different time periods in some of the ASEAN countries. Primary consumption information complements food availability data, since the latter describes average food supplies at the national level, while the former provides an insight into actual dietary intakes at the household level. The present report encountered a scarcity of recent consumption data for a few ASEAN countries.

Patterns of Staple Food Consumption

Cereals. Rice holds the central place among the staple foods and is considered the staff of life throughout ASEAN and in many other parts of Asia. It is common for the people, particularly the poorer population, to derive the bulk of their calories from carbohydrates. In a dietary survey undertaken in 1982 using food weighing method, Konjing and Veerakitpanich [26] found the per capita calorie consumption of the rural families in the Northeastern provinces averaged 2,100 cal per day compared to 1,800 cal consumed by slum dwellers in Bangkok. Cereals, predominantly rice, accounted for 82% of the total calorie intake in the Northeast and 51% in Bangkok. A similar rural-urban pattern of food consumption prevails in Malaysia. In a series of studies carried out in 1979–1983 covering 550 households living in poor villages in different parts of peninsular Malaysia, Chong et al. [10] found that rice and wheat products (flour, bread and biscuits) constituted 61% of the villagers' daily intake of 1,874 cal. In East Malaysia (Sabah), an extensive nutritional study conducted in 1978–1980 revealed that the Kadazan and other natives settled on upland areas and coastal plains had 70–74% of their calorie intake from cereals, rice mainly [8]. By comparison, urban households in the Peninsula were found to rely less on cereals for calories (52% of the total) [28].

Due to the bulk of cereals in the diet, the poorer people in ASEAN derive a major proportion of their protein from cereals. Lie et al. [27] reported in 1976 that plant foods contributed 63–82% of the total protein consumed by Indonesians from different islands. In Maluku and Irian Jaya, for example, the staple plant foods comprised of rice and maize (mainly), sago and sweet potato. The amount of cereals in the Filipino diet makes it the dominant contributor of many nutrients besides protein. In 1978, Villavieja [40] found the one-day per capita cereal intake of 334 g in Luzon and Visayas contributed 54% of total protein, thiamine and niacin intakes. Furthermore, 40 and 34% of iron and riboflavin intake respectively were obtained from the cereal group.

Fish and Livestock Products. Besides cereals, fish occupies an important position in supplying protein to the ASEAN people. Fresh or salted fish is practically the sole animal protein among the lower income families in Indonesia ranging from 27.3 g per person per day in Jawa to 3.3 g in Kalimantan [27]. In the Philippines, fresh, dried, smoked and processed fresh water and salt water fish amounted to 67 g per capita per day [40]. Among Malaysian villagers, fish consumption is high as revealed in a number of studies [10, 44]. The daily quantity of fish eaten averaged about 70–100 g per capita in the inland villages compared to over 100 g in coastal locations. In this manner, 25–35% of the total protein came from fish and seafood. A similar level of fish protein constituted the diet in Singapore in 1978 [2].

In general, consumption of meat is low when compared to fish. Religious prohibitions on pork by Muslims and on beef by Hindus and Buddhists result in poultry meat being probably the most popular meat of the various races in the ASEAN region. The demand for livestock products tend to increase with income as reflected by their higher consumption among the more affluent. Among the urban households in Malaysia, the consumption of meat (including poultry), eggs and milk was found to be 2.4, 1.9 and 1.6 times respectively more than that in the rural sector [28]. The contribution of these three items to the total protein consumed in rural areas was 12% only [10]. Likewise, in the rural Northeastern provinces of Thailand, the people had less protein of animal origin than their urban counterparts [26]. Meat and eggs contributed 17 and 31% of the rural and urban consumption of animal protein respectively. Milk is largely an imported item in the ASEAN countries and, hence, it is outside the reach of the lower income group. In Metropolitan Manila, daily per capita intakes of milk as well as of eggs, meat and poultry were 2–2.5 times greater than those in the rural parts of Luzon – Visayas [40]. Sweetened condensed milk was the preferred type of milk reported in these surveys, whereas fresh fluid milk is taken at an insignificant level. Under 2% of 1,219 households in urban-rural locations in Malaysia included fluid milk in their daily diet [44].

Food Availability versus Consumption Data

Intakes of calories, protein and fat, as obtained from some nutrition surveys, are compared with food balance sheet data for the corresponding periods. The comparison is restricted only to Thailand and Malaysia since more recent survey data could be obtained for these two countries. In both countries, available calories per capita per day was reported to be higher than the levels obtained from surveys (table 14). A difference between the

Table 14. Comparison of available calories, protein and fat with consumption levels (per capita per day)

	Calories		Protein		Fat	
	available calories[1]	consumption of calories[2]	available protein[1], g	consumption of protein[2], g	available fat[1], g	consumption of fat[2], g
Malaysia	2,549		58.0 (24.9)[3]		56.9	
Rural		1,988		48.8 (20.0)		26
Urban middle class		2,162		62.0 (32.0)		32
Thailand	2,322		45.9 (12.2)		28.4	
Rural		2,125		63 (15)		15
Urban slums		1,777		57 (27)		59

[1] Period for available calories, protein and fat: Malaysia and Thailand, 1982–1984.
[2] Survey period: Malaysia, 1986 [28]; Thailand, 1982 [26].
[3] Grams of animal protein in parentheses.

two sets of data is expected, reflecting food wastage, overeating by the affluent and inherent problems in collating and analyzing data on a per capita basis [36]. The gap is widest among the poor, be they in rural villages or urban slums. In Malaysia, rural consumption of calories was 22% below the availability average, while the urban areas had 15% less. The problem is made more acute by the fact that these poverty populations had consumption levels of energy below the recommended daily allowances. In 1982, the rural poor in Malaysia had a calorie intake which ranged between 79 and 101% of the recommended level.

It was found that the rural Northeastern region of Thailand had a comparatively higher calorie intake than the urban slums. Both groups belong to the lower income sector; however, the subsistence farmers in the Northeast do not have to rely as much on purchases as the urban households, being able to derive the bulk of their calorie needs from their own cultivation of rice, cassava and maize. In comparing with availability data, the calorie consumption by the Northeastern region amounted to 91.5% of the national average, whereas the slums showed an intake level of 76.5% only (table 14).

With respect to protein intake, dietary surveys found its level close to or higher than the national availability figures for Malaysia and Thailand. Malaysian urban households consumed more protein, including animal protein, than their rural counterparts. In Thailand, it is the rural region that recorded a higher level of protein intake than the urban slums in Bangkok; however, the latter's intake of animal protein was found to be greater, indicating that the rural Northeastern region tends to derive most of its protein from rice and other plant sources.

In comparing fat consumption with its availability, it was found that both the rural and urban households in Malaysia did not consume as much fat as reported in its food balance sheet. In contrast, the urban sector of Thailand showed fat consumption to be twice the national average, whilst its rural region had an intake of approximately one quarter of that consumed by the urban households.

Trends in Food Trade

The role of food trade is considered to be of major importance in relieving supply deficits in developing countries. In 1976–1980, all the four developing regions of Asia, North Africa/Middle East, Sub-Sahara

Africa and Latin America were net food importers [33]. In Asia, imports of basic food staples, mainly cereals, were about double its exports in the late 1970s. Paulino [33] also pointed out that between 1966–1980, net food imports in East and Southeast Asia increased by about a million tons in a decade. The present report found that ASEAN as a group managed to remain a net exporter of food in the early 1980s. This is due to the largest two exporters in this group, namely Thailand and Malaysia, showing a positive annual export growth during 1980–1983 (table 15). Brunei Darussalam was the other member to produce a positive growth but her export volume was miniscule in relation to that of the other members. On the other hand, the decreasing rate of food exports shown by Indonesia and the Philippines may reduce ASEAN's position as a net exporter. Singapore's negative rate of exports reflects a decline in her entrepot food trade, rather than a reduction in food production.

In 1983, food imports contributed 15.6% of total imports for Brunei Darussalam, the highest proportion in the region, followed by 10.7% for Malaysia. These two countries also showed the fastest increase rate for food imports between 1980 and 1983 (at 13.7 and 5.1% respectively). Thailand depended least on food imports which amounted to only 3.8% of

Table 15. Food[1] imports and exports: ASEAN countries, 1980–1983 [18]

	Food imports in 1983 million US$	Food exports in 1983 million US$	Average annual change 1980–1983, %		Food imports ÷ total imports in 1983, %	Food imports ÷ total exports in 1983, %
			imports	exports		
Brunei Darussalam	113.2	4.0	13.7	23.9	15.6	3.3
Indonesia	1,247.2	1,284.0	−1.4	−4.3	7.6	5.9
Malaysia	1,414.7	2,196.2	5.1	4.3	10.7	10.0
Philippines	573.4	1,490.3	4.0	−9.5	7.7	9.8
Singapore	2,098.6	1,351.1	2.0	−4.4	7.5	9.6
Thailand	394.7	3,228.7	−2.5	11.4	3.8	6.2
ASEAN (total)	5,741.8	9,554.3	–	–	–	–

[1] Food and animals + beverage + oilseeds + animal and vegetable oil + fish and fishery products.

her total. Moreover, her import of food has been decreasing at 2.5% per year. The food bill for the other three member nations averaged 7.5% of their total imports.

A country's food imports can also be considered in terms of the proportion of foreign exchange earned through total exports which has to be spent on importing food. The gap between export earnings and food expenditure at the macro level can be over 100% in critical food deficit countries where demand for imports climbs as production falls. In ASEAN, food imports ranged from approximately 3–6% for Brunei Darussalam, Indonesia and Thailand, to about 10% for the Philippines, Singapore and Malaysia. Brunei Darussalam is actually a net importer of virtually all her food needs, but due to huge exports of crude oil, natural gas and petroleum products (a total of US$ 7 billion in 1984), her food import pales on comparison.

Table 16 highlights the net trade of some major foods of ASEAN, showing that in 1984 the region was a net exporter of rice, maize, sugar and palm oil. Besides these commodities, ASEAN also ranked as a net exporter of fruits, such as bananas, pineapples and mangoes, coffee, cocoa beans, pepper, cassava and coconut products including copra, coconut oil and

Table 16. Net trade[1] of major food items in ASEAN in 1984 [5, 18]

	Rice		Maize	Wheat[3]	Meat[4]	Milk[5] and cream	Sugar	Palm oil
	1980	1984						
	1,000 MT[2]		1,000 MT	1,000 MT	10 MT	10 MT	10 MT	1,000 MT
Brunei Darussalam	−16	−17	−0.1	−5	−511	−358	−760	−1
Indonesia	−2,012	−414	+101	−1,452	+14	−108	−31	+228
Malaysia	−168	−438	−953	−552	−2,388	−4,602	−44,353	+2,551
Philippines	+263	−190	−182	−778	−214	−5,528	+88,031	−28
Singapore	−188	−210	−318	−160	−6,495	−4,229	−12,379	−9
Thailand	+2,798	+4,616	+3,116	−141	+3,384	−4,199	+124,020	−3
ASEAN (total)	+677	+3,347	+1,562	−3,088	−5,986	−10,626	+154,528	+2,738

[1] Net trade is exports minus imports: plus for net export and minus for net import.
[2] Metric tonnes.
[3] Wheat + flour.
[4] Fresh, chilled or frozen.
[5] Evaporated, condensed, dried or fresh.

desiccated coconut [5]. In this respect, Thailand plays a significant role in being solely or largely responsible for ASEAN being a net exporter or rice, maize, cassava and sugar, among other food exports. Rice is a case in point where all the ASEAN countries in 1984 were net importers, with the exception of Thailand (table 16). Between 1980 and 1984, the net trade for rice increased fivefold due mainly to a 65% increase in rice export by Thailand and a corresponding 79% decline in its import by Indonesia. However, the Philippines and Malaysia increased their reliance on rice import over the same period by 1.7 and 2.6 times respectively. Malaysia has reviewed downward its target for self-sufficiency in rice to vacillate between 55 and 65% from a previously targeted level of 85% [41].

With regards to maize, Thailand recorded over 3 million metric tonnes for export in 1984. The other ASEAN exporter of maize is Indonesia who, until 1983, was a net importer because of its high yielding seed varieties that provided for profitable production being persistently damaged by disease (downey mildew). The country's production has improved tremendously and in 1984 she managed to export about 100,000 metric tonnes. Malaysia is a leading ASEAN importer of maize for food and currently 95% of its import comes from Thailand.

Thailand and the Philippines were the only exporters of sugar among the ASEAN countries in 1984 (table 16). However, the position of the latter as a net exporter of sugar has become precarious because, not only is the country badly hit by the slide in sugar price since the early 1980s, resulting in the fall in cane production and closure of mills, but the Philippines is also embroiled in a recently decreed land reform aimed at dividing up the sugar haciendas among the millions of the landless poor. Sugar exporters around the world are already encountering very stiff competition, made worse by a sugar market that has been diminishing since 1982 [21]. The Food and Agriculture Organization estimates that since 1973, developed countries have decreased the annual per capita sugar consumption by 5 kg or 12%, especially among net importers of raw sugar, notably the USA, Canada and Japan. Health implications from excessive sugar intake is believed to be partly responsible for the cutback in these countries.

Malaysia provided the major proportion of the palm oil trade in ASEAN, with Indonesia contributing about 8% to the region's net export of 2.7 million metric tonnes in 1984. Malaysia relies on palm oil and products for 18.6% of her total export earnings in 1984 [5]. Dependence on a few primary commodities for export has resulted in Malaysia being subjected to the vagaries of changes for these commodity prices. As an exam-

Table 17. Relationship between per capita income and imports of selected higher valued food items [18]

	Gross national product per capita in 1984, US$	Average growth rates of real gross domestic product, 1971–1984, %	Per capita imports (kg) in 1984		
			meat[1]	milk[2]	wheat[3]
Brunei Darussalam	not available	4.5	23.7	6.0	2.4
Indonesia	490.9	7.1	0.02	0.3	9.0
Malaysia	2,004	7.6	1.6	4.9	39.5
Philippines	602	4.7	0.05	1.0	14.6
Singapore	7,139.2	8.8	28.3	14.1	79.8
Thailand	801	6.5	0.01	0.9	2.9

[1] Fresh + chilled + frozen meat.
[2] Dry milk.
[3] Wheat + fluor in wheat equivalent.

ple, the price of palm oil averaged about US$ 450 per tonne in 1985, but plummeted to below US$ 200 by March 1986.

The ASEAN region in 1984 was a net importer of wheat, meat, milk and cream. Population growth and rising incomes in the region are propelling the demand for these higher-valued food items. Brunei Darussalam, buoyed by one of the highest per capita GNP in the world, imported substantially more livestock products on a per capita basis than the rest of ASEAN in 1984, with the exception of Singapore (table 17). A major percentage of Brunei's meat import comprised of duck meat (41.7%), while beef, beef preparations and veal constituted approximately 24% of its total meat import, followed by chicken meat at 14.2% [15]. As for Singapore, her per capita imports of meat, milk and wheat products were 28.3, 14.1 and 79.8 kg respectively. About two thirds of Singapore's meat import was for chicken meat (64.1%) followed by mutton and lamb (11.6%) and pork (9.4%) [15]. Singapore also recorded a relatively high level of per capita import of wheat and wheat products. The other ASEAN countries showed comparatively lower per capita import of meat, as pork and chicken meat are produced domestically in adequate quantities to meet the demand of a wide section of the population in these countries. Nonetheless, it has been postulated that the import for beef will rise as its demands has been growing at the estimated rate of 5–6% in Thailand [38] and Malaysia [41].

Nutritional Implications

Population Increase and Food Production

Between 1961 and 1980, Asia (excluding China) increased production of major food crops by 2.8% yearly, and it is projected that she will increase at an average annual rate of 3.0% between 1980 and 2000 [33]. In comparison, ASEAN as a group performed almost twice as well with food production showing yearly increase of 5.4% between 1970 and 1979 (table 18). In 1980–1984 the region's annual increase rate of 3.0% was closer to the projected figure for Asia in general. While food production continues to increase, so does population growth. In Asia (excluding China), population expanded by 2.4% per year between 1961 and 1980. Consequently, food output on a per capita basis increased at a minuscle level of 0.1% for Asia (excluding China) during the 1960s and 1970s [33].

The annual growth rate of population varies widely among the ASEAN countries, ranging from 1.2% for Singapore to 3.9% for Brunei Darussalam between 1980 and 1984; the average growth rate for ASEAN during the same period was 2.4%, which is similar to the rate for Asia (table 18). Population growth in ASEAN is at a comparable level with the average rates of other developing regions such as Latin America (2.6%) and North Africa/Middle East (2.7%) [33]. During the past 20 years, the

Table 18. Annual growth rates (%) of population and food production[1] in ASEAN [4, 18, 33]

	Population		Food production		Per capita food production	
	1970–1979	1980–1984	1970–1979 (1969–1971 = 100)	1980–1984 (1974–1976 = 100)	1971–1979 (1974–1976 = 100)	1980–1984 (1974–1976 = 100)
Brunei Darussalam	3.5	3.9	–	–	–	–
Indonesia	2.3	2.2	3.2	3.5	1.5	0.6
Malaysia	2.4	2.6	5.1	3.7	2.2	0.7
Philippines	2.8	2.5	3.9	0.9	3.0	-0.7
Singapore	1.5	1.2	9.1	6.8	10.2	4.4
Thailand	2.5	2.0	5.8	4.2	1.8	1.0
ASEAN	2.5	2.4	5.4	3.8	3.7	1.2
Asia	2.3 (excludes China)[2]		2.8	4.7	–	–

[1] Food production represents disposable agricultural production for any use except seed and feed.
[2] 1960–1980.

ASEAN nations have experienced an increase in population growth mainly due to the reduction in mortality rates. Family planning programs have had a limited impact on reducing birth rates, with the exception of Singapore, where its success, especially in the 1960s and 1970s, is closely due to national social policies [7]. Under conditions of relatively high population growth rates, food production is hard-pushed to stay abreast of demand.

Table 18 shows that between 1970 and 1979, food production growth exceeded population increase in all the ASEAN countries. This pattern prevailed in 1980–1984, with the exception of the Philippines whose production rate fell behind its population growth rate. In general, the food growth rates for all the ASEAN countries were higher during the 1970s (averaging 5.4%) than between 1980 and 1984 (3.8%).

When food production is expressed on a per capita basis, it brings into focus the reality that food growth in ASEAN has been insignificant throughout the 1970s, and even less encouraging in the first half of the 1980s. The average per capita food production change for ASEAN was 1.2% per year between 1980 and 1984, with Indonesia, Malaysia and Thailand averaging 1.0% or less annually. The Philippines recorded a negative per capita index during this period. Such a slow rate of growth seems to indicate very little improvement in the nutritional status of the population in general and among the poor in particular.

Prevalence of Malnutrition

One of the most common forms of malnutrition in this region is protein energy malnutrition (PEM), particularly among growing children. Table 19 shows the magnitude of PEM in Indonesia, Malaysia, the Philippines and Thailand. Albeit that different classification of PEM had been used, the prevalence of mild to moderate type was identified in fairly high percentages. In Indonesia, 30% of the preschool children were estimated to be affected by mild to moderate PEM. This compares with 15.8% in the Philippines having moderate PEM. In Thailand, 6.7% of the infants and school children were assessed to show moderate PEM. It was found that among poor preschoolers in rural Malaysia, 37% were underweight and 43% stunted. Almost as high a prevalence of stunting and underweight was shown by children 6–12 years old in Malaysian villages.

Aside from PEM, iron-deficiency anemia and vitamin A deficiency also pose as important health concerns in different parts of ASEAN. Anemia was recognized in approximately one third to half of the preschool children in Indonesia, Malaysia and the Philippines (table 20). In Thailand

and Malaysia, 30–60% of school children were shown to be anemic. Among pregnant women, a higher proportion extending to 70% was examined to be at the anemic level. Vitamin A deficiency in the form of xerophthalmia is the most important cause of blindness in Indonesia [39]. It was estimated that 3–4 per thousand or about 100,000 preschool children become blind each year. Vitamin A deficiency is not such a serious public health problem in the rest of ASEAN.

Iodine deficiency resulting in goiter tends to be localized in its prevalence. Endemic areas, such as the mountainous interior of Sabah and Sarawak in East Malaysia, and the rural North and Northwestern regions in Thailand, have a high percentage of the population, especially among the women, with iodine deficiency goiter (table 20).

Table 19. Prevalence of PEM in ASEAN [39]

	Indonesia 1980–1981	Malaysia 1979–1983	Philippines 1984	Thailand 1985
Preschool children	30% mild to moderate 3% severe	43% stunted 5% wasted 37% underweight	15.8% moderate 2.2% severe	(infants and school children) 28.5% mild 6.7% moderate 0.8% severe
Children 6–12 years	–	49% boys and 35% girls stunted 2% boys and 2% girls wasted 38% boys and 23% girls underweight	–	(school children in rural areas) 14–42% mild 1–7% moderate

Classification of PEM:
Indonesia: Mild to moderate PEM is 60–80% Harvard standard of body weight for age. Severe PEM is below 60% Harvard standard.
Malaysia: Stunting is height for age below –2 standard deviations of the National Centre for Health Statistics (NCHS) median. Wasting is weight for height below –2 SD of the NCHS median. Underweight is weight for age below –2 SD of the NCHS median.
Philippines: Moderately malnourished is 60–90% below the Philippines' growth standard of body weight for age. Severely malnourished is below 60% of the Philippines' growth standard.
Thailand: Mild PEM is 75–89% of Thailand's standard of weight for age based on modified Gomez's classification. Moderate PEM and severe PEM are respectively 60–74% and below 60% of Thailand's standard.

In contrast, the young children in Singapore have been found to manifest the consequence of overnutrition. Between 1976 and 1983, a total of 705,511 school children aged 7–12 years were screened for obesity based on the Quatelet's index [23]. It was revealed that the prevalence of childhood obesity reached 8% of the boys and girls in 1983, and is on the increase. This is a reflection of the growing affluence of the country, whose demand for total calories, protein and animal fats has been on the rise, as shown previously by the food availability data.

It is recognized that food consumption is closely correlated with the GNP of a country, but what is more important nutritionally is available income for food at the household level. Geissler and Miller [19] found malnutrition to be more prevalent in the Philippines than in Thailand, despite the considerable rise in GNP over the last decade in both countries. The critical difference lies in the higher inflation rate in the Philippines,

Table 20. Prevalance of anemia, vitamin A deficiency and goiter in ASEAN [39]

	Indonesia 1980–1981	Malaysia 1979–1983	Philippines 1982	Thailand 1985
Iron deficiency anemia				
Infants	–	34%	50%	–
Preschool children	40%	33%	32% (preschool and school children)	10–40%
School children	9%	37% (adolescent girls)	–	30–60%
Adults	–	25% (18–45 years female)	–	17–37%
Pregnant women	70%	–	49%	30–70%
Vitamin A deficiency				
Preschool children	50% with night blindness	–	1.8% with night blindness 1.4% with Bitot's spot	–
Iodine deficiency goiter	10–90% endemic areas	1.5% of total population in Sarawak; endemic in Sabah and Northern Peninsular Malaysia	7.6% women of child-bearing age, 7.5% lactating mothers, 3.2% pregnant women in endemic areas	10% school children in North and Northeast regions

Iron deficiency anemia:
Malaysia: less than 15% serum transferrin saturation.
Thailand: less than 33% hematocrit level.

thereby rendering its cost of basic needs including food to be higher than in Thailand. Although income data from household surveys should be interpreted with caution, nonetheless, the persistence of malnutrition in the region serves to indicate that there exist certain segments of the population, who are too poor to afford nutritional adequacy for their children and pregnant and lactating women. The proportion of such poverty-stricken communities varies from country to country in the region, with Singapore and Brunei Darussalam perhaps least afflicted on account of the absence of a poor rural sector, as is found in the other member countries.

While the plight of the rural poor has long been recognized, countries are only recently coming to grips with the health problems of urban squatters. Between 1970 and 1980, the proportion of urban to total population increased by 5% in Indonesia, which is equivalent to 12.1 million people. During the same period, the urban population increase in Malaysia was 7.4% (13.8 million), in the Philippines, 4.4% (5.6 million), and 3.8% (3.1 million) in Thailand [37]. A comprehensive health and nutritional study on spontaneous settlements in Manila in 1975 identified 9.6% of the population from 6,000 households to have third-degree malnutrition, 37.5% of them showing second-degree malnutrition, and 20% with anemia [6]. Within any city, there are some slum areas which enjoy a higher nutritional sufficiency than others, as demonstrated in a study of ten squatter communities in Bangkok in 1982 [26]. The calories index ranged from 55 in one location to 130 in another (a nutrient index of 100 indicates adequacy), while that for protein and iron was found to range between 69 and 253 and between 100 and 385 respectively.

One consequence of rural-urban migration on food production is that the agriculture labor force becomes reduced. Between 1973 and 1983, the population in the agriculture sector decreased by 4–5% in Thailand and the Philippines, and by 8–9% in Indonesia and Malaysia [35]. Rice fields, rubber and oil palm plantations in Malaysia encounter a shortage of workers, and so labor has to be contracted from countries such as Indonesia. With a rapid rate of population growth, Indonesia's population has reached 168 million in 1987. In order to reduce the population in high-density Java, transmigration was conceived and since 1950, hundreds of thousands of families have been re-settled, particularly in Sumatra, followed by Kalimantan. Cash crop cultivation on larger holdings is emphasized in order to improve the standard of living of the transmigrants [3]. Marketing and other problems abound with the transmigration program, and consequently, able-bodied men have sought employment elsewhere.

Concluding Remarks

ASEAN became 20 years old in August 1987, and its claim to international prominence has been greater in the field of politics, especially in respect of its efforts to reconcile the disparate groups in Kampuchea, than in regional economic collaboration as originally envisaged for the organization. Differences in national economic priorities remain deep and it has been suggested that the similarity in factor endowment and climatic conditions among the member countries has resulted in their economies becoming more competitive than complementary [9]. Intra-ASEAN trade in 1985 amounted to less than one fifth of the group's trade with the rest of the world. Individually, each of them has forged ahead averaging 4.5–9% annual growth in real gross domestic product between 1971 and 1984 [18]. In respect of food production, ASEAN as a group manages to export a variety of important foodstuffs including rice, maize, cassava, sugar, fish, poultry, fruits, palm oil, beverages and spices.

However, this enviable food situation in ASEAN needs to be considered in the light of two caveats. Firstly, the group owes its net food export position mainly to just one member country, namely Thailand. The remaining members are net importers of food including rice (with the exception of Indonesia). Secondly, the high population growth rate of the group (except for Singapore) will not help to ameliorate the problem of inequitable distribution of food. Although food availability data indicated that the average national supply of calories and most nutrients were adequate, the persistence of PEM as well as the deficiencies of iron and vitamin A in parts of ASEAN demonstrates the ironical manifestation of hunger amid a region of plenty. A high population growth also tends to negate improvements in food production and the countries will rely increasingly on food imports to meet the growing demands. Malaysia, as an example, imported US$ 260 million worth of food items in 1975, but the bill totalled an astronomical US$ 1.4 billion in 1984. The need to reduce food imports has become imperative in view of the substantial losses in export earnings from primary commodities, whose prices plunged during 1985–1986.

Since large segments of the population in ASEAN depend upon agriculture, it is socially and politically rational for ASEAN to strive for regional food security in the long run. Towards this end, not only rice but other food staples should be included in the effort to coordinate supply, stock piling and food trade. ASEAN already has established a multitude of projects with foreign assistance (for example, Australia, the USA, Canada and Japan) for technical cooperation and development in many areas of agriculture such as food handling, plant quarantine training, seed technology, forest management and agriculture cooperatives. Success in regional integration of agricultural production and trade would further boost ASEAN's economic standing in the world.

Acknowledgements

The authors would like to thank Dr. Rahmat Qureshi, Regional Food Policy and Nutrition Officer of the Food and Agriculture Organization Regional Office for Asia and the Pacific, for his kind assistance in obtaining the unpublished FAO Food Balance Sheets for 1982–1984. We would also like to thank Mr. W.K. Wong of the Photography and Medical Illustrations Unit of the Institute for Medical Research for preparing photographs of all the illustrations.

References

1 Abe, T.: Changes in nutritional allowance for the Japanese. Asian med. J. *29:* 249–259 (1986).
2 Ang, H.G.; Lim, K.K.; Theng, C.Y.: Food eating habits in Singapore; in Bayan, Valdecanas, Proc. 1st ASEAN Seminar-Workshop on Food Habits, Manila 1978, pp. 75–100 (ASEAN Sub-Committee on Protein, Manila 1978).
3 Arndt, H.W.: Transmigration: achievements, problems, prospects. Bull. Indonesian Econ. Stud. *19:* 50–73 (1983).
4 ASEAN Selected Statistics 1967–1984 (ASEAN Secretariat, Jakarta 1986).
5 ASEAN Statistical Yearbook on Food, Agriculture and Forestry 1978–1984 (ASEAN Agricultural Development Planning Centre, Bangkok 1986).
6 Basta, S.S.: Nutrition and health in low income urban areas of the third world. Ecol. Food Nutr. *6:* 113–124 (1977).
7 Chang, C.T.; Ong, J.H.; Chen, P.S.J.: Culture and fertility: the case of Singapore (Institute of Southeast Asian Studies, Singapore 1980).
8 Chen, P.C.Y.; Chan, M.K.C.; Teoh, S.T.; Bent, B.; Yap, S.B.; Fong, T.; Ong, F.P.T.; Lee, M.C.C.: A nutrition study of the Interior, West Coast and Kudat Divisions of Sabah (University of Malaya, Kuala Lumpur and Office of the Director of Medical Services, Kota Kinabalu 1981).
9 Chew, E.F.C.: ASEAN cooperation in agriculture. Options *2:* 6–8 (1987).
10 Chong, Y.H.; Tee, E.S.; Ng, T.K.W.; Kandiah, M.; R. Hanis Hussein; Teo, P.H.; Siti M. Shahid: Status of community nutrition in poverty kampungs (Institute for Medical Research, Kuala Lumpur 1984).
11 Danielson, R.; Robbins, L.: Food consumption trends in Canada – the last 20 years. Food Market Commentary *6:* 47–57 (1984).

12 De Boer, A.J.: Livestock development: the Asian experience, in Fine, Lattimore, Livestock in Asia. Issues and policies, pp. 13–26 (International Development Research Centre, Ottawa 1982).
13 FAO Food Balance Sheets 1975–77 Average and Per Caput Food Supplies 1961–65 Average, 1967–1977 (FAO, Rome 1980).
14 FAO Food balance Sheets 1979–81 Average (FAO, Rome 1984).
15 FAO Food balance Sheets 1982–84 Average (FAO, Rome, unpublished).
16 FAO Production Yearbook, vol. 36 (FAO, Rome 1982).
17 FAO Production Yearbook, vol. 38 (FAO, Rome 1984).
18 FAO Trade Yearbook, vol. 38 (FAO, Rome 1984).
19 Geissler, C.; Miller, D.: Nutrition and GNP. A comparison of problems in Thailand and the Philippines. Food Policy *7:* 191–206 (1982).
20 Girardot-Berg, I.: Livestock: policy issues in trade, pricing and marketing; in Fine, Lattimore, Livestock in Asia. Issues and policies, pp. 91–96 (International Development Research Centre, Ottawa 1982).
21 Haris, S.: Current issues in the world sugar economy. Food Policy *12:* 127–145 (1987).
22 Herdt, R.W.; Capule, C.: Adoption, spread and production impact of modern rice varieties in Asia (International Rice Research Institute, Manila 1983).
23 Ho, T.F.: Childhood obesity in Singapore primary school children epidemiological review and anthropometric evaluation. J. Singapore Paed. Soc. *27:* 7–40 (1985).
24 Human Monitoring Division, Human Nutrition Information: Nationwide food consumption survey: continuing survey of food intakes by individuals – 1985. Nutr. Today *May/June:* 18–22 (1986).
25 Jarvis, L.S.: To beef or not to beef? Portfolio choices of Asian smallholder cattle producers; in Fine, Lattimore, Livestock in Asia. Issues and policies, pp. 29–41 (International Development Research Centre, Ottawa 1982).
26 Konjing, K.; Veerakitpanich, M.: Food consumption and nutrition in Thailand; in Panayotou, Food policy analysis in Thailand, pp. 157–187 (Agricultural Development Council, Bangkok 1985).
27 Lie, G.H.; Hermana; Sumardi; Siti Isnijah: Food consumption patterns and food habits in Indonesia. Proc. 1st ASEAN Seminar-Workshop on Food Habits, Manila 1978, pp. 34–41 (ASEAN Sub-Committee on Protein, Manila 1978).
28 Mohd. Ghazali, M.; Siti Khairon, S.: Food availability and patterns of food intake. Proc. Seminar on Food Security and Policy Issues (Universiti Pertanian Malaysia, Serdang, in press).
29 Mohd. Mahyuddin, D.: Livestock production: status, constraint and prospect. Proc. Seminar on Food Security and Policy Issues (Universiti Pertanian Malaysia, Serdang, in press).
30 Mubyarto: The sugar industry: from estate to smallholder cane production? Bull. Indonesian Econ. Stud. *13:* 29–44 (1977).
31 Palm Oil Research Institute Malaysia (Ministry of Primary Industries, Kuala Lumpur 1985).
32 Panayotou, T.; Puapanichya, K.: Output supply and input demand in rice and upland crop production: the quest for higher yields in Thailand; in Panayotou, Food policy analysis in Thailand, pp. 23–94 (Agricultural Development Council, Bangkok 1985).

33 Paulino, L.A.: Food in the third world: past trends and projections to 2000 (International Food Policy Research Institute, Washington 1986).
34 Qureshi, U.A.: Current concerns in nutrition in the Asia-Pacific region. Proc. 2nd Scientific Conf., Kuala Lumpur 1987 (Nutrition Society of Malaysia, Kuala Lumpur, in press).
35 RAPA Monograph: 1985/8. Agriculture in Asia-Pacific – a pictorial profile (Regional Asia-Pacific Association, FAO, Bangkok 1985).
36 Scrimshaw, N.S.; Lockwood, R.: Interpretation of data on human food availability and nutrient consumption. Food Nutr. Bull. *2:* 29–34 (1980).
37 SEAMIC Health Statistics 1986 (Southeast Asian Medical Information Center, Tokyo 1986).
38 Tokrisna, R.; Panayotou, T.: An overview of the livestock sector in Thailand with special reference to buffalo and cattle; in Fine, Lattimore, Livestock in Asia. Issues and policies, pp. 130–137 (International Development Research Centre, Ottawa 1982).
39 Tontisirin, K.: Travel Research Followship survey findings on the nutrition situation and action programs for improvement in SEAMIC countries (Southeast Asian Medical Information Center, Tokyo 1985).
40 Villavieja, G.M.: A food consumption profile in the Philippines; in Bayan, Valdecanas, Proc. 1st ASEAN Seminar-Workshop on Food Habits, Manila 1978, pp. 48–74 (ASEAN Sub-Committee on Protein, Manila 1978).
41 Wan Ibrahim, W.D.: Food policy; the government perspective. Proc. Seminar on Food Security and Policy Issues (Universiti Pertanian Malaysia, Serdang, in press).
42 Wawn, B.: The economies of the ASEAN countries (Macmillan, Hongkong 1982).
43 Wong, J.: ASEAN economies in perspective (Macmillan, Hongkong 1983).
44 Zanariah, J.; Yunos, J.; Rosnah, O.; Nor Rehan, A.: Studies of the food intake trend of the population in urban and rural areas in four selected districts in West Malaysia (Malaysian Agriculture Research and Development Institute, Serdang 1985).

Geok Lin Khor, PhD, Department of Human Development Studies,
Universiti Pertanian Malaysia, 43400 Serdang (Malaysia)

Bourne GH (ed): Aspects of Food Production, Consumption and Energy Values.
World Rev Nutr Diet. Basel, Karger, 1990, vol 61, pp 41–63

Bioconversion of Urban and Agroindustrial Residues into High Quality Protein Through Aquaculture

Newton Castagnolli[1]

Faculdade de Ciências Agrárias e Veterinárias UNESP, Campus de Jaboticabal, S.P., Brazil

Contents

Introduction

Hundreds of millions of people around the world coexist with the grim specter of hunger [54]. Vieira-Gallo [64] states that almost 500 million human beings – 10% of humanity – are suffering hunger and 40 thousand children die every day for reasons directly linked to calories, protein or vitamin deficiency. Considering these aspects Kinne [24], at the World Conference on Aquaculture held at Venice, confirmed that the production of food for those millions of people remaines a serious problem.

[1] I would like to thank Mr. Deusimar Freire Brasil and Márcio Adriano Favero for their secretarial and editorial assistance.

The FAO's task is a constant fight against universal hunger, especially in the rural areas of developing countries.

Van der Wal [61] states that we need new food resources and should not restrict ourselves to increasing supplies of existing sources to meet the increasing demand. In our attempts to develop these potentials we should avoid theoretical overkill. The author mentioned that there are 9,000 million ha of land in the world. Around 50% of this area consists of forests and shrublands. Another 35% is pasture and grasslands and only 15% is arable land; the major part of the produce grown on arable land is discarded as residue. Food science and technology at present concentrate mainly only on the 5% of the annual production of the potential nutrients that can be used after relatively simple forms of processing such as cooking or baking. This means that the 95% that is not yet utilized directly for human consumption needs a considerable processing, be it physical, chemical or via some bioconversion form before it can be turned into suitable feed or food.

At the FAO's Technical Conference on Aquaculture held at Kioto, Japan, during the opening ceremony, Pillay [40] stated that aquaculture could be increased by 5 or 6 times – from 5–6 million metric tons produced at that time to 25–30 million tons produced all over the world at the end of this century if national governments, especially those of tropical countries, made serious efforts in order to develop aquaculture programs starting by manpower capacitation at all levels.

In order to achieve this goal the various factors of production and their interplay must be studied in order to establish appropriate steps for both vertical and horizontal integration of the operative enterprises. There is still a need of strong and well-oriented governmental inputs, especially those for the first financial and technical supports at the onset of the aquaculture activity in the farm since fish production is the cheapest way to obtain high-quality protein, but there is a relatively high capital requirement for the construction of the rearing facilities [17].

According to Webber and Riordan [66] it is expected that the world aquacultural production will exceed the present value of the total capture before the end of this century. Although the affirmation of those authors may be considered rather optimistic, it is interesting to note that Robinson [42] considered that since the demand for fish food could double in the next 20 years while trends in production looked like remaining less dynamic, the tendency would be an increase in the price of fish. Thus, the growth of fish production in the developing countries during the last decades had not been sufficient enough to prevent the drastically declining rate of growth of the world total catch – from 5 to 1 % per year in the 1970s – due to the diminishing of the stocks of the conventional fish that suffer overcatches continuously with the progress in capture technics.

In our understanding, aquaculture is the shortest way to increase fish production to levels the upper limits of which are quite impossible to estimate.

Recycling of agricultural and agroindustrial wastes and their bioconversion into food for direct or indirect (through domestic animals) human consumption is based mainly on taking the best profit of the 'free of charge' solar energy and its use in many ways in order to reduce the production costs of food which may enhance a production in sufficient amounts in order to solve or at least to reduce the world's major problem of human hunger.

The United Nations have declared 1986 as the 'International Year of Peace'. The FAO on the 'World Food Day (October 16)' has published a paper by Vieira-Gallo concerning on 'The Right to Food – a Contribution to Peace', in which the author discusses the problem of hunger in the world linked to the right to food, a basic human right without which the right to life is in itself meaningless. The fulfillment of the right to food is viewed as an irreplaceable contribution to the maintenance and consolidation of peace.

Article 11 of the International Convenant on Economic, Social and Cultural Rights is probably the most judicious source of the right to food because it recognizes the right of everyone to adequate food and freedom from hunger.

The real problem we have to recognize is that although there exist the amendments – and the Declaration of Human Rights is a rich source – the real difficulty is their accomplishment and the fact that there is no punishment for those who are in fault with them.

But even considering that in most of the cases the problem of hunger is more a political than a technical task, humankind can easily remove the Malthusian ghost of universal hunger through application of technological advances in crop and animal husbandry production associated with many biotechnological combinations of algal, aerobic and/or anaerobic microorganisms for waste treatments with production of single cells proteins (SCP) that may be used for food in animal husbandry and/or aquaculture. The latter one, that involves less energy costs, may be considered the new frontier for food production and so far the true way to start the 'blue revolution', through which the recycling of agroindustrial wastes or the integration with animal husbandry and agriculture, especially in tropical areas – where the poverty is more acute – has an important role to play in order to reach this goal.

Biological Basis of Aquatic Bioconversion

According to O'Brien and de Noyelles [36], one of the earlier and most important contributions of limnology to fish culture was Brant's observation in 1899 that N and P are the aim-limiting nutrients for primary production in freshwater environments.

Zeller [71] observed through daily chemical (phosphorus levels) and biological (plankton production) tests that there is a good correlation between the concentration of phosphates and plankton production in Missouri (USA) farm ponds. The author also stated that the phosphate is confined to the bottom by a stable summer stratification.

Hepher [20] observed that ponds fertilized with ammonium sulfate and simple superphosphate yielded five times higher primary production – expressed in mg $C/m^2/h$ – when compared with nonfertilized ones. Hepher [21] agreed with this affirmation stating that P (PO_4^{-3}) dissolved in the water is usually low, hence most of the P remains adsorbed to the bottom coloids or to other organic suspended particles.

Russel-Hunter [43] showed that N is more promptly assimilated as nitrates (NO_3^-) and is eliminated as organic N through the continuous excretion of live aquatic organisms or definitively by their death. The organic N is rapidly recycled by the action of decomposing nitrificant bacteria to ammonium (NH_4^+), nitrites (NO_2^-) and nitrates (NO_3^-).

Smith and Swingle [52] were the first researchers who made correlation studies between fish and plankton production in fertilized and nonfertilized ponds in Auburn, Alabama.

According to Schindler and Fee [46], Birlinsky, in the same year, found that the primary production is highly correlated with latitude; this means that light and temperature are really important factors in stimulating the organic (primary, secondary and fish) production in ponds, lakes and reservoirs.

Effectively, Nasar and Datta-Munshi [34] conducted a one-year primary production study in a permanent freshwater pond at Bhagalpur, India (25°15′ N lat.) and they observed that the net primary production in

April (the month with the highest temperature) was 7 times greater than observed in September.

Castagnolli [8, 9] observed a 70% higher fish production during summer as compared to that obtained during the same period (60 days) in winter, in the same ponds stocked with the same amount of fish – common carp and nile tilapia. The 12 ponds had received the same type and amounts of organic (rabbit manure) and mineral NP, N or P in Jaboticabal, São Paulo State, Brazil (22° 25′ S lat.).

McFadyen [30] made a description of the structure of the natural biological communities that are based on competition between organisms feeding on the same resources and on the 'layering' of the community which results from the feeding habits of different species and is represented by the Eltonian dynamic cycle.

Thus, the eutrophication of freshwater ponds combined with polycultural rearing of fish (several fish species with different and noncompetitive feeding habits) enhances increments in primary and fish production through the optimization of energy transfers between the nearest steps (trophic levels) of the food webb.

Zur [72] has carried out the determination of primary productivity, water respiration and other biological and chemical parameters in earthen experimental ponds. The ponds were stocked with common carp or tilapia hybrids in a monoculture at stocking rates varying from 7,000 to 20,000 carp and 20,000 to 100,000 tilapia/ha. The fish biomass was up to 23 ton/ha. The primary productivity was higher in the ponds with higher stocking rates within the same species and higher in the carp ponds than in those stocked with tilapia.

The author calculated a complete carbon balance for each pond summing up all the sources of inputs and outputs of carbon in the pond and calculated the surplus that grew with the increasing fish densities up to 8,900 kg C/ha per year in the ponds stocked with 20,000 carp/ha.

Oláh et al. [37] concluded that fish production efficiency varied over a wide range both in temperate or tropical lakes or reservoirs (ponds), the average fish conversion being more efficient in temperate regions. This conversion efficiency depends on many factors, such as the methodologies employed, fish species involved, stocking density, nature of fertilizer and intensity of the ponds.

Noriega-Curtis [35] also carried out studies of various parameters associated with periodicity in experimental manured ponds with the objective of estimating the effects of manure application and fish yields. Net photosynthetic rates were found to be only slightly higher than those obtained under chemical fertilization. Their variation seemed to be independent of the total standing crop of the plankton and more closely related to composition of the plankton. Several fish yield prediction models based on primary productivity applied to experimental data showed that the obtained productions considerably exceeded the predicted yield which means that fish production does not always depend on primary productivity.

Aquacultural Technics

Integration of Aquaculture with Animal Husbandry and Agriculture

A broad study of marine natural productivity in terms of total catches shows that it had been maintained almost constant – around 65–70 million metric tons – in the last decade. The most optimistic expectations suggest that this figure can probably be increased by a further 20–30 million metric tons if a better exploitation of pelagic species is combined with an increase in fishing efforts. Even so there is a limit for the natural productivity in the oceans and inland waters and the harvest through fishing boats or any other fishing device is always an extractive and increasingly expensive activity due to the pollution of natural environments that causes a serious reduction in fish stocks and moreover results in higher fishing efforts and energy expenditure in order to obtain the same amount of fish.

Torloni [59, 60] states that in the underdeveloped countries there is a shortage of inorganic fertilizers; the use of organic wastes, including domestic sewage, should be recommended, and it is already used in overpopulated countries like China and India.

The development of adequate technologies for each tropical area where the use of agricultural and industrial residues, locally produced, that may convert into high quality protein through aquaculture, as the Chinese already have done for centuries, may double or even further increase the fishery production which is now around 75–80 million metric tons, including capture and aquaculture. Besides that, an improvement is needed in the utilization of the fish harvested from the sea since around 20% of the catches never reaches the consumer; thus, they are lost on their way to market or are usually delivered to produce fish meal for animal consumption.

Another important consideration is that the natural productivity of freshwater fisheries is highly dependent on man's intervention in the environment, such as the construction of dams for electric power generation, irrigation of rural areas or urban water supplies, and pollution by industrial and domestic effluents or pesticides; the tendency is a constant and sharp decline in wild catches.

Aquaculture seems to be the only way to overcome these constraints and the recycling of urban and industrial effluents is, without any doubt, the most economic and advantageous way.

Bardach and Santerre [3] stated that the use or organic residues in aquaculture can either be extensive with wastes occurring naturally or being added with little or no further management for production or it can be highly intensive under conditions where extraneous feeding is supplied every day. The authors state that many compilations in the literature allow quantitative comparisons of fish yields under various conditions of more or less intensive regimes in temperate regions and they are always inferior to those obtained in the tropical areas.

The production of vertically integrated aquaculture to agriculture and animal husbandry may attain higher levels when different fish species are stocked in fertilized ponds, especially if supplementary feed is added to the fish ponds. The way Chinese farmers have been able to obtain high rates of production from traditional fish farming is based on a polyculture of compatible species of Chinese carps, which is effectively done by judicious combinations of silver carp and big-head carp which feed on plankton and generally occupy the surface water, grass carp and 'wuchan fish', which are herbivores, feed on grasses and vegetables and occupy mostly the middle layers of the ponds and common carp and black carp that live on the bottom and feed on detritus or benthic organisms. This polycultural rearing system is further consortiated with pig or chicken/geese cultures with rational utilization of the rations.

According to the FAO [15] China, besides its great tradition, has one of the highest potentials for aquaculture. The country has some 20 million ha of freshwater areas and at least one third is suitable for fish farming; from this at least 1.3 million ha is now under some form of cultivation. The FAO/UNDP mission that had visited China in 1979 mention that not only the ponds are used for fish farming; larger bodies of water, such as natural lakes, reservoirs, canals and small rivers, are also used for fish cultivation. Collective ownership has made feasible the management of much larger water areas for fish farming in which more than 20 species are cultivated in fresh and brackish water.

Annual fresh and coastal water fish production is around 2.5 million tons and for that some 20 thousand million fry of freshwater fishes are produced and distributed all over the country. On a country-wide basis production is reported to be 800–900 kg/ha/year in open waters and 4–5 tons/ha/year in ponds.

The FAO mission concluded that two main factors are responsible for such impressive but realistic production figures: the tradition of Chinese people to produce and to eat fish and the government policy in organizing the management of fisheries within the country through planning, extension work, credit and financing and also the adoption of more recent fish culture practices including artificial propagation or induced breeding technics.

Oláh et al. [37] studied the fish yields in ponds under different management practices comparing the efficiencies of energy conversion from primary levels to fish production obtained in temperate conditions in Hungary with the yields of the tropical undrainable, rural fish ponds of Orissa, India. The authors observed in Hungary productions of ponds only stocked, others that received only inorganic (20 kg N + 150 kg P) fertilization and others fertilized with domestic sewage at a rate of 100 m^3/ha and pig manure at a rate of 2 m^3/ha. In all of these observations fish were stocked in spring and harvested 6 months later (autumn).

The authors observed a higher fish conversion efficiency in the ponds only stocked with the fish but production in the fertilized ponds were doubled when compared with the nonfertilized ones. They concluded also that there is no close relationship between primary production and fish production. The same may be said from the results obtained in Orisa where the highest daily fish production (15.8 kg/ha) was observed in a pond with low primary production.

In the Philippines, Grover and Banacia [18] might be the pioneers in trying polyculture of three carp species ('rohu' – indian carp – common and silver carp). They mention production five times higher in the fertilized ponds as compared to the unfertilized ones.

At that time Woynarovich [68] started, in Hungary the preliminary attempts on the feasibility of combining fish farming with animal husbandry, with reference to duck and pig production.

In Brazil, Sobue et al. [53] made the first attempts on the use of organic manure associated with mineral (N or P) fertilizers studying in 1973 the biotic productivity of the fish ponds of Jaboticabal's Agrary Sciences Faculty stocked only with common carp and, in the North-Eastern region of Brazil, Da Silva et al. [11] developed the first trial-consortiating swine to fish culture and demonstrated that fish culture associated to the recycling of organic residues (piggery wastes) is a very profitable protein production system and an important way to reduce the pollution in the earth. Besides that in such a warm region (very low latitude) and alkaline soils fish in the fatening ponds present high growing rates throughout the year. Indeed they have obtained 3 tons/ha/year of fish (hybrid tilapia) stocked at a density of only 5,000 fingerlings per hectare.

Lovshin and Malca [29] mention that in Panama fish producers are instructed to build tilapia reproduction and nursery ponds along with a large grow-out pond that are associated with chicken, pig, duck or cattle operations. Vegetable gardens, fruit and pine trees complete the integration, enhancing a high and continuous fish supply throughout the year.

Aguilar studying the feasibility of rearing tilapia in a swine waste lagoon recommended a stocking rate of 25 hogs/acre of lagoon stocked with 1,200 fingerlings per acre, which for us seems to be a high stocking rate for hogs and low fish density in the pond.

Buck et al. [6] had probably been the first Nort-American researchers who made consortiation studies between swine and fish culture, trying a polyculture rearing of common and other Chinese carps, with native species such as black bass, channel catfish and 'hybrid buffalo'. The authors produced around 3,000 and 3,800 kg/ha in the ponds where it was raised – 40 and 66 animals/ha of pond fish culture.

Stickney et al. [56] conducted a trial in ponds stocked with 6,000 *Tilapia aurea* with the following treatments: (a) control; (b) 210 laying hens/ha; (c) 220 hogs/ha; (d) 74 hogs/ha, and 25 hogs/ha. Poultry and swine were maintained over the ponds in suspended cages and slotted floor respectively, to allow waste products and spilled feed to fall directly into the water. The authors observed rapid growth of *Tilapia aurea* in the ponds receiving chicken waste and the two lowest levels of hog waste. The poorest growth of the fish was observed in the pond with 220 hogs/ha and a complete kill of the fish was observed in the ponds receiving the intermediate level of hog waste just before the termination of the experiment, probably due to a complete water quality deterioration with the coverage of the pond surface with duck weed.

Lili et al. [27] have conducted a fertilization trial in 3 ponds of 0.06 ha stocked with 30 pairs of the blue tilapia *(Oreochromis aureus)* broodstock (males weighing 400–500 g and females 170–350 g each). The ponds were manured with three different rates (equivalent to 64.4, 47.4 and 27.2 kg/ha/day of swine manure). Tilapia standing stock harvested after 90 days ranged 44 kg/ha in the medium manure rate pond, to 320 ka/ha in the low manure rate pond.

McGeachin and Stickney [31] stocked 50 all-male *Tilapia aurea* in 7-m^2 plastic pools which received direct input of laying hen manure at the rate of 0, 35, 70 or 140 kg dry weight per hectare/day during 1978 and 70, 140, 210 or 280 kg dry weight per hectare/day during 1979. On the basis of growth and survival of the blue tilapia and water quality data obtained suggest that the manuring rate in summer should be between 70 and 140 kg of laying hen dry manure per hectare/day, depending on the alkalinity of the water, meaning that the lower end of the range should be when the alkalinity of the water is high.

Zhang et al. [70] studied the ecological effects of varying the sizes of fish ponds loaded with manures and feed, stocking the ponds with Chinese carp species, such as grass carp, big-head carp, silver carp, common carp, crucian carp, and 'wuchang' fish. Aquatic grass was given as supplementary feed for grass carp.

Two trials during 200 days each were conducted in 1982 and 1983 using 9 ponds of different sizes, from 1 'mu' (667 m^2) to 11 'mu' (7,333 m^2). Dissolved oxygen was lower in the smaller ponds. The average yield attained 6,090 kg/ha. The conversion rate of pig manure and aquatic grass on fish biomass was 17:1 and 85:1, respectively. The best size of fish ponds that enhanced higher fish yields were between 3.0 and 5.7 'mu' (1,999–3,800 m^2).

There was no direct relationship between primary productivity, organic detritus and fish yields. The same was found to occur between the nutrient levels of total nitrogen, ammonia, nitrite and phosphate and the fish yields.

Almost all of the fish stocked attained marketable size at the end of the experiment which showed a good total stocking density of 15,000 fish/ha in 1982 and 18,000 fish/ha in 1983 at the following proportions (fish/ha): 1982, 7,500 silver carp; 1,550 bighead carp; 4,500 grass carp; 1,500 common carp; 1983, 4,500 silver carp; 3,000 'wuchang' fish; 3,000 crucian carp and the other species as 1982.

Watson [65] tested anaerobically digested piggery waste as a substitute protein source at 10 and 20% levels on an isonitrogenous and (as far as possible) isocaloric basis and compared it to a control diet of soybean meal and fish meal for fingerling mirror carp *(Cyprinus carpio).* The fish fed on the substitutive diet showed significantly higher ($p < 0.05$) specific growth rates; the fish on the 20% piggery waste diet had significantly lower ($p < 0.05$) fat contents and significantly higher ($p < 0.05$) ash contents compared to both the control and the 10% diet. The author observed that raw animal wastes do not perform well when substituted for conventional protein sources in fish diets.

There remains in an almost virgin state a great potential to fish culture in tropical countries with the 'domestication' of wild promising South American fish species, mainly those belonging to Colossoma and Brycon, Characidae from the Amazon river basin as suggested by Saint-Paul and Werder [44] or even other species of the Parana-Uruguay river basins, such as Prochilodus and Piaractus (= *Colossoma mitrei*), species that have already been propagated through induced breeding technics, and a few million fingerlings are annually produced in Brazil, Venezuela and Colombia.

Use of Domestic Sewage in Aquaculture

Bailly [2] has developed a trial concerning the polycultural rearing of fish in ponds supplied with domestic effluents from a sedimentation lagoon. The water presented high nitrogen and phosphorus concentrations which enhanced high primary (algae) and secondary (animal microorganisms) production. Different fish species (Chinese carps) with different feeding habits were stocked in the ponds. Fish biomass production without any supplementary feeding was 2.6 tons/ha.

According to Schroeder and Hepher [47] cow manure and sewage from small towns are quantitatively demonstrated to be commercially useful bases for natural fish foods. Cow manure applied at daily rates of 200–1,000 l/ha/day as fish biomass increased from less than 500 kg/ha to greater than 4,000 kg/ha and resulted in fish yields of 20–40 kg/ha/day with no use of supplementary feed. Intensive manuring in conventionally fed fish ponds resulted in doubled yields of fish with half the usual feed requirement.

The authors report that in Israel the sewage from a town of 5,000 inhabitants fed directly into a 4-ha reservoir-pond yielded 2,800 kg fish/ha/6 months with no supplementary feeding and sewage from a 500-person kibbutz, fed into 3 ha of fish ponds which received supplemental feeds, yielded 8,600 kg fish/ha/8 months, as compared to 4,700 kg/ha/8 months in adjacent ponds not receiving sewage.

Use of Industrial Wastes, Heated Effluents and Recirculation Systems

Shelef [50], discussing the project set up at the Haifa Institute of Technology, suggests that the principal bioregenerative process involves the intensive growth of algae on wastes with emphasis on its combination with anaerobic bacterial processes. Pond fish can be associated to the bioregenerative scheme or even another less well established biological system, such as nitrogen fixation by the blue green alga *Anabaena azolla* which is symbiotically associated with Azzola fern in rice paddies replacing commercial nitrogenous fertilizers.

According to Shelef [50] all biological processes involved in the bioregenerative concept are well established in nature's cycles of organic matter degradation and primary productivity, and in the food chain. Within the bioregenerative farm they have intensified this process manyfold, increasing the biomass productivity by optimizing the physical conditions and the growth-limiting factors, such as substrate and nutrient concentrations, light intensities (in the case of algae), retention time, etc.

Stanton [55], analyzing the possibilities of bioconversion of fruit and vegetable wastes, considered that people from many regions of the world have developed ingenious methods of fermentation to overcome inherent indigestibility or toxicity of the protective (fruit-skin constituents) and not-to-be-eaten components of plants by a combination of physical (to destroy the anti-microbial factors) and microbial methods that act to dispose of alkaloids, glycosides (CN- and S- compound-containing), phenolics, saponins, sterols, toxic peptides and anti-enzymatic factors, to name the most commonly found compounds inhibiting consumption.

Fruit residues, such as wastes from manufacturing plants that process fruits for juice extraction or sweet production, may be used directly or after cooking in carp pond fish-rearing unities – like the Santa Catarina fish farmers using apple-skins or the people from the Vale-do-Ribeira region in São Paulo State who use banana coats, enhancing substantial increments in fish yields. In this case the pond acts like a biodigestor and develops high populations of fermentative bacteriae – the SCP – that, once eaten with the decomposing fruit material, increase the protein content of the natural cheap food.

In Japan, according to Ebine [14], at the beginning of the 1970s, there was a strong research effort on industrial production of SCP obtained from agro-wastes, involving investigations on methods to assess the safety, feed value, and acceptability of SCP products as well as the means to pelletize and store the produce.

The main agro-wastes considered for the production of SPC were soybean cooking waste, cellulosic residue from saw mill waste, rice straw and rice husks, citrus wastes and fish-processing wastes, and the microorganisms utilized for SPC production were *Aspergillus orizae,* Candida sp., Saccharomices sp. and Tricoderma sp.

One of the major problems faced at that time by Japanese researchers was the high chemical oxygen demand (COD) of soybean cooking waste, and they were trying mechanical, chemical and biological methods for the reduction of this high COD.

Tacon [58] conducted a detailed chemical and nutritional analysis of activated sludge single cell protein (ASCP) from samples collected at biweekly intervals from rural workers' domestic sewage during one year. The analysis revealed that the ASCP present a nutritive value broadly equivalent to brewer's yeast or a protein-rich cereal.

Effectively the author has conducted a series of combinatory nutrition trials incorporating ASCP up to the level of 33% to pelleted trout diets (on an isonitrogenous and isocaloric basis) and concluded that ASCP can easily replace soybean meal and wheat middlings up to a level of 33% in terms of growth response and food conversion of the fish that did not present any toxic or carcinogenic effects during the trials.

Van Weerden [62], considering the nutritional value of the four categories of microorganisms involved in bio-conversion processes (yeasts, bacteria, fungi and algae), states that there is only a limited amount of information available concerning the nutritional value of yeasts.

The author mentions that in order to make a complete evaluation of the nutritive value of a product, many trials need to be conducted in a sequence that is finally recommended for animal and/or human consumption. Trials involve primarily a bromatological analysis of its nutrients, such as protein, fat, ash, carbohydrates and preferably also the amino acid contents.

The second step includes acceptability studies in order to determine whether the inclusion of a moderate or high dose of the test product in the diet affects feed intake (palatability), and complete digestibility trials may indicate the energy values (metabolizable and/or digestible energy). The last trial should be a comparative feeding experiment in which the test product replaces partially or all the usual high protein components in the diets in order to see how it affects weight gain, egg production, feed conversion efficiency and product quality.

Bressani [5] states that from the total amount of energy devoted to agricultural production only a small fraction is harvested to be used direct or indirectly for animal and human consumption. Most of the energy is left behind in the field, in food processing factories or lost – eaten by insects or mice during storage processes. So care must be taken in order to avoid such tremendous losses.

The author also reminds the reader that the evaluation of bioconverted products to be used as food must take into account four main problems: toxicology, public health aspects, food technology and nutritional quality.

The nutritional quality of the byproducts such as algae (Chorella) or SCP such as Torulla or yeast may be evaluated through nitrogen intake (g/day), nitrogen balance (g/day) and protein digestibility determinations. SCP are the nongaseous products from bioconversion of organic residues.

Another important consideration is that once nontraditional food sources begin to be utilized for human consumption it becomes necessary to establish the guidelines for their safety.

Lewis et al. [25] designed a closed fish production system maintaining the water quality by the use of biofilters and tanks for hydroponically grown vegetables. The biofilters facilitated the digestion of ammonia, feces and waste feed to a mineralized form, especially nitrates. The biofilters floculated a large amount of suspended solids. In the hydroponic culture additional biofiltration occurred in the gravel beds and the plants removed the nitrates and phosphates. The authors [26] later improved the design to maintain water quality by biofiltration and plants grown hydroponically arranged in a way to give reciprocating water flow without the use of elevated reservoirs, and they concluded that this system is applicable to a closed system of seed fish and may prove attractive for private or commercial production of food fish and vegetables, especially in regions that suffer shortage of good quality water. This system also presents the great advantage of producing vegetables without the use of fertilizers.

Ferreira and Schoonbee [16] used a storage pool for cooling water from a stream-electric power generating plant in Johannesburg, South Africa. Most of the water is obtained from a continuous supply of treated domestic sewage effluent discharged into the pond at a rate of 18–36 m^3/day. The pond was stocked with tilapia (*Oreochromis mossambicus* and *Tilapia rendalli*) and the Chinese silver carp *(Hypophthalmichthys molitrix)*. Pond water temperature fluctuated from 21 to 30 °C which, with the high nutrient loads, enhanced frequent algal blooms and extended the breeding period for tilapia, leading to stunting in the growth rate. Even so, more than 3 tons of fish yearly has been removed by seine netting.

Hilge [22] developed a trial aiming at the possibility of establishing a commercial fish farm using a closed warm-water system in the Federal Republic of Germany. The author developed a growth curve model in order to optimize the stocking rates and stocking sequences in relation to the final mean body weight of fish for the given total capacity of a 50-m^3 circuit enhancing the production from 1.5 to 8.6 tons of fish/year obtained when using a semi-monthly stocking sequence of mirror carp. In cases like this or other similar race-ways coupled to recirculation systems, it may enhance higher productivity but always with high energy (feed and cost) imputs which are not feasible for the underdeveloped tropical and subtropical countries.

Meske [32] describes an experimental method of keeping, feeding and propagating warm-water food fish in a closed and heated water system independent of climatic influences and environmental pollution. In this rather sophisticated rearing technic, effluent from fish tanks passes into an aerated activated sludge tank where aerobic microorganisms decompose the protein-containing sludge particles in the waste water. Nitrifying bacteriae oxidize nitrogenous excrements and feed residues to ammonium nitrogen and then to nitrite and nitrate. The sludge next flows into a sedimentation tank without aeration where it settles to the bottom. Denitrification takes place here under anaerobic conditions where nitrogen is set free and the gas escapes, so the purified water continues through a heating and pumping tank and back to the fish tanks.

Behrends and Smitherman [4] had described a method that enhances rearing Tilapia spp. in temperate countries even during winter months in order to get off-season spawnings in aquaria supplied with a continuous flow of condenser cooling water from nuclear power plants that kept the aquaria water temperature around 14 °C above the ambient water sources. Spawning occurred at least 60 days ealier than in the controls and enhanced a fast growing of the fingerlings during spring and summer and the production of marketable tilapia ($>$ 250 g) in a single growing season.

Degani et al. [12] found that digested slurry may substitute partially high protein content diets for tilapia *(Oreochromis niloticus),* enhancing a similar performance with a significant reduction in the cost of production.

Coche [10] – summarizing many papers presented at the World Symposium held at Stavanger, Norway from 28th to 30th May 1980 on 'Aquaculture in Heated Effluents and Recirculation Systems', sponsored by EIFAC/FAO (European Inland Fisheries Advisory Committee of the Food and Agricultural Organization of the United Nations) – mentions that the symposium aimed the discussion at the use of heat from both natural and industrial sources, the methods for an efficient use of water, including recirculation systems, and tried to identify areas that required further research as well as recommending the action to be taken in this field.

In the symposium many recommendations arose concerning water quality requirements related to chemical characteristics, such as dissolved oxygen, ammonia, nitrates, pH, alkalinity, chlorine, etc., or physical ones, like color, transparency suspended solids and conductivity, seeking to obtain water conditions that may enhance greater productivity, via efficient monitoring of pond water quality.

A serious constraint with the use of heated effluents and recirculation systems is the gas supersaturation that may lead to fish stress and predisposition to infectious diseases, most of them of rather difficult solution.

Considering such problems the symposium recommended: (1) The effects of fish culture facility effluents on natural fish populations should be studied. (2) Engineering consultancy on ponds and facility construction and also water quality monitoring through constant chemical analysis. (3) Biological aspects must be also considered, such as the choice of fish species resistant to the accumulation of metabolites in water and the suitability for intensive culture combined with the study of the best use of natural and artificial warm-water resources in order to reduce production costs, thus making the fish production unit feasible. For sure such high-priced rearing systems are only feasible for temperate climate, developed countries or in places where the water is a limiting factor; hence it is possible to maintain high stocking densities in ponds at an average water temperature of 23 °C, enhancing the growth within one year of common carp and European catfish from the egg stage up to 1.5–2.5 kg.

Constraints to Wider Applications

Modern societies are forced to use water supplies that contain a large amount of water previously used by man, i.e. 'waste waters' [1]. The authors state that the use of waste products to fertilize ponds can increase the growth and production of fish and, on the other hand, fish may improve the waste treatment capacity of pond systems.

According to Webber and Riordan [66] the problems of large-scale integrated aquaculture are: species limitations (in the market, biological and technological); site selection; manpower needs, and legal, institutional and financial requirements and, for a new future, if we consider aquaculture as a growing industry seed supply, disease control and water quality will have to be improved in order to maintain a steadily increasing slope of continuous increments in fish yields.

Allen and Hepher [1] add that restraints on waste-water fish culture include: unsatisfactory dissolved oxygen levels in ponds; presence of toxic materials in waste waters; presence of unacceptable tastes and odors in fish (off-flavor); various problems of public health; difficulties of satisfying pond effluent standards; meeting public acceptance of the practice.

Allen and Hepher [1] conclude that waste-water aquaculture requires much information on an understanding of many processes, especially those concerning the physico-chemical dynamics of pond environment in relationship to the physiological requirements of the cultivated species and suggest that there is a need of a cooperative interdisciplinary approach in order to solve the actual difficulties of the integration of aquaculture, agriculture and public health.

According to Scrimshaw [48], many products obtained from plant and animal residues, although technologically viable and economically feasible, have had to be abandoned because of unacceptable additional costs for the elimination of hazards or because of regulatory or political obstacles. The author also mentions that fears had been related to the organisms produced in such processes which, even if normally nontoxic, might undergo mutation to toxic strains or become contaminated by toxic ones. Concern also focused on the possible carry-over of toxic substances from substrates to SCP intended for direct human consumption or into products for human consumption from animals fed on these materials. In Japan, for instance, due to an erroneous research report, the production of SCP became a political issue, and this has blocked all efforts to use this product even for animal use.

According to Schacklady [45], toxicological evaluations present, in general, three problems. The first is inherent in the science itself; the others are related to the nature of the material to be evaluated and the circumstances in which its use is contemplated. The inherent problem exists regardless of the type of product of its intended use and can be stated in very simple terms. The problem associated with the nature of the material relies on the fact that classical evaluation procedures were not developed with bioconversion products in mind.

The third type of problem, concerning the circumstances in which a material may be used, can be subdivided into two parts. One is related to the practical and the other concerns the ethical or philosophical considerations on the use of the products.

The feeling is that absolute safety does not exist. The question remains on the balance between the risk attendant upon the use of products and the benefit that would accrue. This ratio will vary according to the circumstances: what might be acceptable in one case may be quite unacceptable in another. Substances from normal domestic sewage and the costs of such separation systems will ultimately influence the feasibility of their use.

Bardach and Santerre [3] also state that one of the constraints to wider application of organic manures in fish culture is, to a certain extent, dependent on competition for these residues by agricultural systems. On the other hand, sewage utilization in aquaculture is conditioned by cultural, sanitary and economic constraints in which they agree with Scrimshaw [48]. Disease and parasite transmission, while still a consideration, are often overrated when the sewage of small or large towns is used for aquaculture. The presence of industrial wastes may be potentially hazardous from the standpoint of toxic substances that accumulate in the flesh of the fish and the use of such wastes for the production of food for humans should be allowed only when it is possible to segregate these toxicants (toxic substances).

Another important item related to the acceptability of the wastes for human consumption is the aspect and palatability that will require advanced technological processing in rather sophisticated plants; these will require high amounts of funds for their construction.

Last but not least it is necessary to include an economic approach in these comments upon the bioconversion of wastes into protein. Slesser [51] stated that the energy costs in a flow-through biological system must not only be considered as a monetary aspect but as a comparison of all energies involved in a production system in order to use the least energy that enhances the production of the same amount of biomass.

Conclusions

The bioconversion of urban and agroindustrial residues into high quality protein – fish meat – through aquaculture that, besides reducing the production costs of food, represents an important way of eliminating the pollutant wastes of urban and rural communities. In other words, this seems to be as well as the 'Columbus egg', an important key in solving two enormous problems that afflict us with growing intensity every year with the constant growing of the earth's population: universal hunger and what to do with the byproducts of human activities.

In order to focus on so wide a range of interdisciplinary problems, considerations were made on the biological basis of aquatic bioconversion, the aquacultural technics involving the integration of aquaculture to animal husbandry and agriculture, the use of domestic sewage and industrial wastes in aquaculture, including heated effluents and the possibility of recirculation systems where water shortage may occur, including the legal, institutional and medical aspects of the use of the fish produced through these recycling systems and obviously the constraints that may arise and limit the wider applications of the aquatic bioconversion of the abovementioned residues.

From what had been pointed out there is no doubt that mankind is en route to dominating all the technological problems of producing sufficient amounts of food to face the Malthusian ghost of universal hunger through this 'blue revolution', producing food in a not new but not yet well-explored frontier: the fresh, brackish and marine waters. There are two important characteristics of water bodies: one intrinsic of water as a universal solvent, and the other (extrinsic) is the low energy cost of photosynthesis as a bioconversion agent of the wastes into high quality food.

References

1 Allen, G.H.; Hepher, B.: Recycling of wastes trough aquaculture and constraints to wider application. FAO Tech. Conf. on Aquaculture, Kyoto 1976. FIR: AQ/Conf./76.R/19: 18 p. (pre-prints).

2 Bailly, J.M.: Essais d'aquaculture en effluent de lagunage. Symp. on Finfish Nutrition and Fish Feed Technology, Hamburg 1978. EIFAC/78/Symp.: E/29: 30 p. (pre-prints).

3 Bardach, J.E.; Santerre, M.T.: Organic residues in aquaculture. Bioconversion of organic residues for rural communities. Food Nutr. Bull., suppl. 2, pp. 72–83 (1979).

4 Behrends, C.C.; Smitherman, R.O.: Use of thermal effluents in tilapia hatchery management. Prog. Fish Cult. *14* (1985).

5 Bressani, R.: Nutrition evaluation in humans. Bioconversion of organic residues for rural communities. Food Nutr. Bull., suppl. 2, pp. 160–166 (1979).

6 Buck, D.H.; Baur, R.J.; Rose, C.R.: Experiments in recycling swine manure in fish ponds. FAO Tech. Conf. on Aquaculture, Kyoto 1976. FIR: AQ/Conf./76. E/29: 5 p.
7 Camara-Dantas, L.: Ponte dos Carvalhos experiment with tilapia: a case study on land and water mismanagement and technology transfer (Abstract). Int. Symp. on Tilapia in Aquaculture, Nazareth 1983, p. 99.
8 Castagnolli, N.; Oliveira, G.T.; Ostini, S.; Pereira Filho, M.: Influências da estação do ano e do fertilizante aplicado na produção orgânica de tanques de criação de peixes. I. Produção primária. B. Inst. Pesca, 9 (único): 91–108 (1982).
9 Castagnolli, N.; Camargo, A.F.; Oliveira, G.T.; Ostini, S.: Influência da estação do ano e do fertilizante aplicado na produção orgânica de tanques. II. Produção secundária ede peixes. B. Inst. Pesca, 9 (único): 109–123 (1982).
10 Coche, A.G.: Report of the Symposium of new Development in the Utilization of Heated Effluents and Recirculation Systems for Intensive Aquaculture, Stavanger 1980. EIFAC Tech. Paper No. 39, 37 p. (1981).
11 Da Silva, A.B.; Lovshin, L.L.; Melo, F.R.: Observações preliminares sobre a cultura monosexo da tilápia-do-Nilo, *Tilapia nilotica,* em viveiro, em comparação com híbridos machos de tilápia com o uso de ração suplementat e fertilizante. Proc. Simp. Bras. Alim. Nutrição, 4° Botucatu, pp. 450–451 (1975).
12 Degani, G.; Levanon, D.; Marchain, V.: Substitution of digested slurry (composed of fermented faeces, cow manure, and straw) for *Oreochromis aureus* food. Int. Symp. on Tilapia in Aquaculture, Nazareth 1983, p. 77.
13 Dimitrov, M.: Mineral fertilization of carp ponds in polycultural rearing. Aquaculture *3:* 273–285 (1974).
14 Ebine, H.: Integrated research on agricultural waste reclamation. Bioconversion of organic residue for rural communities. Food Nutr. Bull., suppl. 2, pp. 122–126 (1979).
15 FAO/UNDP.: Aquaculture development in China. ADCP/Rep/79/10: 65 p. (1979).
16 Ferreira, J.T.; Schoonbee, J.J.: Use of heated sewage effluent from a power station for the culture of *Oreochromis mossambicus* and *Hypophthalmichthys molitrix.* Int. Symp. on Tilapia in Aquaculture, Nazareth 1983, p. 101.
17 Gerhardsen, G.M.: Aquaculture and integrated rural development. FAO Tech. Conf. on Aquaculture, Kyoto 1976, FIR: AQ/Conf./76.R/21: 27 p. (pre-prints).
18 Grover, J.H.; Banacia, G.J.: Preliminary yield trial with carp polyculture in fertilized and unfertilized ponds. The Phillipine J. Fish. *11:* 9–22 (1973).
19 Gurgel, J.J.S.: Relatório de Atividades da Diretoria de Pesca e Piscicultura/DNOCS (mimeo) 28 p. (1985).
20 Hepher, B.: Primary production in fish ponds and its application to fertilization experiments. Limnol Ocean *7:* 131–136 (1962).
21 Hepher, B.: Some aspects of phosphorus cycle in fish ponds. Verh. Int. Ver. Limnol. *16:* 1293–1297 (1966).
22 Hilge, V.: Biological and economic aspects of fish production in a closed warm-water system. FAO Tech. Conf. on Aquaculture, Kyoto 1976. FIR: AQ/Conf./76. E/21: 6 p. (pre-prints).
23 Hillbricht-Ilkowska, A.: Secondary productivity in freshwaters; its value and efficiencies in plankton food chain. Proc. 1st Int. Congr. Ecology, The Hague 1974, pp. 164–167.

24 Kinne, O.: Realism in aquaculture. The view of an ecologist. World Conf. on Aquaculture, Venice 1981, 'Reviews' 1–2.
25 Lewis, W.M.; Yopp, J.H.; Schramm, H.L.; Brandenburg, A.M.: Use of hydroponics to maintain quality of recirculated water in a fish culture system. Trans. Am. Fish. Soc. *107:* 92–99 (1978).
26 Lewis, W.M.; Yopp, J.H.; Brandenburg, A.M.; Schnoor, K.D.: On the maintenance of water quality for closed fish production system by means of hydroponically grown vegetable crops. Proc. World Symp. on Aquaculture in Heated Effluents and Recirculation Systems, Stavanger 1980, vol. I, pp. 122–129 (Berlin 1981).
27 Lili, P.S.; Kohler, C.C.; Hausler, C.L.; Arthur, R.D.: Conversion of swine manure into protein feed via Blue Tilapia *(Oreochromis aureum).* Mimeo, 15 p. (1985).
28 Lovshin, L.L.; Silva, A.B. da: Culture of monosex hybrid tilapia. FAO/CIFA/Symp. on Aquaculture in Africa, Accra 1975, SR/9: D/16 p.
29 Lovshin, L.L.; Malca, R.P.: A strategy for the use of tilapias in rural Latin America: The Panamial integrated approach. Int. Symp. on Tilapia in Aquaculture, Nazareth 1983, p. 105.
30 MacFadyen, A.: The meaning of productivity in biological systems. J. An. Ecol. *17:* 75–80 (1948).
31 McGeachin, R.B.; Stickney, R.R.: Manuring rates of production of blue tilapia in simulated sewage lagoons receiving laying hen waste. Prog. Fish. Culturist *44:* 25–28 (1982).
32 Meske, C.H.: Fish culture in a recirculating system with water treatment and activated sludge. FAO Tech. Conf. on Aquaculture, Kyoto 1976. FIR: AQ/Conf./76. E/62: 7 p. (pre-prints).
33 Moav, R.; Wohlafarth, G.L.; Schroeder, G.L.; Hulata, G.; Barash, H.: Intensive polyculture of fish in freshwater ponds. I. Substitution of expensive feeds by liquid cow manure. Aquaculture *10:* 25–43 (1977).
34 Nasar, S.A.K.; Data Munshi, J.: Studies of primary production in a freshwater pond. Jap. J. Ecol. *25:* 21–23 (1975).
35 Noriega-Curtis, P.: Primary productivity and related fish yield in intensely manured fish ponds. Aquaculture *17:* 335–344 (1979).
36 O'Brien, W.J.; de Noyelles, F., Jr.: Relationship between nutrient concentration, phytoplankton density and zooplankton density in nutrient enriched experimental ponds. Hydrobiology *44:* 105–125 (1974).
37 Oláh, J.; Sinha, V.R.P.; Ayyappan, S.; Purushothaman, C.S.; Radaeyshyam, S.: Primary production and fish yields in fish ponds under different management practices. Aquaculture *58:* 111–122 (1986).
38 Pantulu, V.R.: Role of aquaculture in water resource development. A case study of the lower Mekong basin project. FAO Tech. Conf. on Aquaculture, Kyoto 1976. FIR: AQ/Conf./76. E/20 p. (pre-prints).
39 Pillay, T.V.R.; Dill, W.A.: Advances in aquaculture (Fishing News Books, Farnham 1978).
40 Pillay, T.V.R.: State of aquaculture 1981. World Conf. on Aquaculture, Venice 1981. 'Review' (pre-print): 2.
41 Rappaport, U.; Sarig, S.; Bejerano, Y.: Observation on the use of organic fertilization in intensive fish farming at the Ginosar Station in 1976. Bamidgeh *29:* 57–70 (1977).

42 Robinson, M.A.: Prospects of World fisheries to 2000. FAO Fish. Circ. No. 722 (Rev. 1): 16 p. (1982).

43 Russel-Hunter, W.D.: Productividad acuatica, 273 p. (Ed. Acribia, Zaragosa 1973).

44 Saint-Paul, U.; Werder, U.: The potential of some Amazonian fishes for warmwater aquaculture. Symp. Finfish Culture and Fish Feed Technology, Hamburg 1978. EIFAC/78/Symp., E/3: 20 p. (pre-prints).

45 Schacklady, C.A.: Bioconversion products-problems and potential. Bioconversion of organic residues of rural communities. Food Nutr. Bull., suppl. 2, pp. 156–159 (1979).

46 Schindler, D.W.; Fee, E.J.: Primary production in freshwater. Proc. 1st Int. Congr. Ecology, The Hague 1974, Wageningen Centre of Agricul. Publ. and Doc., pp. 155–158 (1974).

47 Schroeder, G.; Hepher, B.: Use of agricultural and urban wastes in fish culture. FAO Tech. Conf. on Aquaculture, Kyoto 1976. FIR: AQ/Conf./76. E/9: 3 p. (pre-prints).

48 Scrimshaw, N.S.: Biomass from organic residues for animal and human feeding. Bioconversion of organic residues for rural communities. Food Nutr. Bull., suppl. 2, 167–170 (1979).

49 Shang, F.L.; Zhu, Y.; Zhou, X.Y.: Studies on the ecological effects of varying the size of fish ponds loaded with manures and feeds. Aquaculture *60:* 107–116 (1987).

50 Shelef, G.: The combination of algal and anaerobic waste treatment in bioregenerative farm system. Bioconversion of organic residues for rural communities. Food Nutr. Bull., suppl. 2, pp. 105–113 (1979).

51 Slesser, M.; Analysis of energy cost of integrated systems. Bioconversion of organic residues of rural communities. Food Nutr. Bull., suppl. 2, pp. 139–143 (1979).

52 Smith, E.V.; Swingle, H.S.: The relationship between plankton production and fish production in ponds. Trans. Am. Fish. Soc. *68:* 309–315 (1939).

53 Sobue, S.; Castagnolli, N.; Pitelli, R.A.: Biotic productivity in fish ponds. Rev. Bras. Biol. *37:* 761–769 (1977).

54 Soedjatmoko: Will mankind be able to secure food in the twenty-first century? Food Nutr. Bull. *7:* 68–71 (1985).

55 Stanton, R.: Bioconversion of fruit and vegetable wastes. Bioconversion of organic residues of rural communities. Food Nutr. Bull., suppl. 2, pp. 120–121 (1979).

56 Stickney, R.R.; Rowland, L.O.; Hesby, J.H.: Water quality *Tilapia aurea* interactions in ponds receiving swine and poultry wastes. Proc. Annu. Conf. World Mariculture Soc., vol. 8, pp. 55–71 (1977).

57 Sutton, R.J.; Lewis, W.M.: Further obversations on a fish production system that incorporates hydroponically grown plants. Prog. Fish. Culturist *44:* 55–59 (1982).

58 Tacon, A.G.J.: The use of activated sludge single cell protein (ASCP) – derived from the treatment of domestic sewage in trout diets. Symp. on Finfish Nutrition and Feed Technology, Hamburg 1978. EIFAC/78/Symp. E/6: 49 p.

59 Torloni, C.E.C.: Reciclagem de resíduos orgânicos na produção econômica de peixes. Aquacultura *1:* 7–8 (1986).

60 Torloni, C.E.C.: Reciclagem de resíduos orgânicos. Aquacultura *2:* 10–13 (1987).

61 Van Der Wal, P.: Perspectives on bioconversion of organic residues for rural communities. Bioconversion of organic residues for rural communities. Food Nutr. Bull., suppl. 2, pp. 3–8 (1979).

62 Van Weerden, E.J.: Nutritional evaluation of bioconversion products for farm animals. Bioconversion of organic residues for rural communities. Food Nutr. Bull., suppl. 2, pp. 152–155 (1979).
63 Venkataraman, G.C.: Indian experience with algal ponds. Bioconversion of organic residues for rural communities. Food Nutr. Bull., suppl. 2, pp. 60–67 (1979).
64 Vieira-Gallo, J.A.; The right to food – a contribution to peace. FAO I/S 2001 (mimeo): 13 p. (1986).
65 Watson, N.R.: Processed piggery waste as a feed material for *Cyprinus carpio*. Aquaculture *44:* 167–176 (1985).
66 Webber, H.H.; Riordan, P.F.: Problems of large scale integrated aquaculture. FAO Tech. Conf. on Aquaculture, Kyoto 1976. FIR: AQ/Conf./76. R/4: 13 p.
67 Wolny, P.: Fertilization of warm-water fish ponds in Europe. World Symp. on Warmwater Pond Fish Culture. FAO Fish Rep. *44:* 64–76 (1967).
68 Woynarovich, E.: The feasibility of combining animal husbandry with fish farming, with special reference to duck and pig production. FAO Tech. Conf. on Aquaculture, Kyoto 1976. FIR: AQ/Conf./76. R/6: 3 p.
69 Yashouv, A.: Mixed fish culture – an ecological approach to increase pond productivity. World Symp. on Warmwater Pond Fish Culture. FAO Fish. Rep. *44:* 258–273 (1967).
70 Zhang, F.L.; Zhu, Y.; Zhou, X.Y.: Studies on the ecological effects of varying the size of fish ponds loaded with manures and feeds. Aquaculture *60:* 107–116 (1987).
71 Zeller, H.D.: Nitrogen and phosphorus concentration in fertilized and unfertilized farm ponds in Central Missouri. Trans. Am. Fish. Soc. *81:* 281–288 (1952).
72 Zur, O.: Primary production in intensive fish ponds and a complete organic carbon balance in the ponds. Aquaculture *23:* 197–210 (1981).

N. Castagnolli, AE, Faculdade de Ciências Agrárias e Veterinárias UNESP,
Campus de Jaboticabal, S.P. (Brazil)

Bourne GH (ed): Aspects of Food Production, Consumption and Energy Values.
World Rev Nutr Diet. Basel, Karger, 1990, vol 61, pp 64–131

Nutritional Needs Assessment of Rural Agricultural Migrants of Southern Brazil: Designing, Implementing and Evaluating a Nutrition Education Program

I.D. Desai[a,b], *A.M. Doell*[a], *S.A. Officiati, A.M. Bianco, Y. Van Severen, M.I. Desai, E. Jansen, J.E. Dutra de Oliveira*[b]

[a] School of Family and Nutritional Sciences, University of British Columbia, Vancouver, B.C., Canada;
[b] Faculty of Medicine, University of São Paulo, Ribeirão Preto, S.P., Brazil

Contents

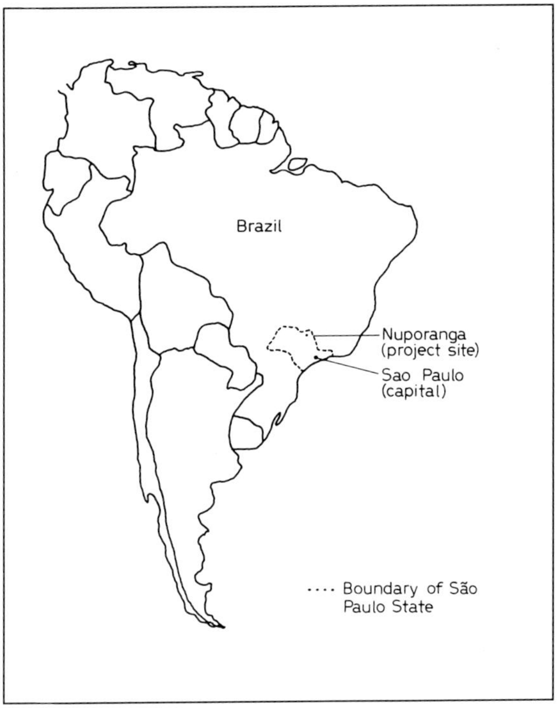

Fig. 1. Map of South America, outlining Brazil, Sao Paulo state, state capital, and project site.

Introduction

Brazil is the fifth largest country in the world and comprises approximately one half the area of the South American continent (fig. 1). The country is divided into 5 major regions (north, northeast, south, southeast, and central-west), 23 states, 3 territories, and 1 federal district [Nyrop, 1983].

Brazil's geography is varied, ranging from coastal plains, savannah, and escarpment to tropical rain forest. Climatic conditions are also varied, ranging from tropical in the north to temperate in the south.

With an estimated population of 125 million in 1983 [Nyrop, 1983], Brazil ranks as the sixth most populated country in the world. The population, however, is unevenly distributed. More than 90% of the population reside in three regions (northeast, southeast, and south), representing less than 35% of the physical area [Roett, 1978].

Portuguese explorers discovered Brazil in the 1500s. Brazil became a Portuguese colony, obtaining its independence in 1822. Although Brazil elected to govern as a republic, the political power remained in the hands of a small elite group [Roett, 1978].

The present military government has been in power since the coup in 1964. Recently, the government has cautiously initiated a more liberal policy in preparation for a possible return to civilian rule. General elections for state and federal representatives were permitted in 1982, the first election since 1964.

Brazil, considered the most industrialized of developing nations, has a population growth rate and age distribution typical of other developing countries. Growth rates in the early 1980s were estimated at 2.47%, one of the highest in South America [Nyrop, 1983]. The age distribution of the population includes a large proportion of young people. In 1980, approximately 48% of Brazil's population was less than 20 years of age [Kluck, 1983]. Other statistics in 1975 indicated that 19% of the population was 5 years of age or younger [Pollitt, 1981].

Brazilian society has been described as a highly stratified class system. One of the primary factors in the differentiation among the various classes of society has been family background. Other criteria, however, such as skin color, wealth, occupation, education, and life-style have also been considered important.

Until the 20th century, Brazilian society consisted primarily of two classes. These classes originated from the large plantations in which the small elite group of landowners provided a paternalistic environment for their workers [Weil et al., 1975; Kluck, 1983].

The structure of society gradually changed as industrialization began in the late 19th century. Industrialization resulted in an increasing number of urban dwellers who would eventually form the urban lower, middle, and upper classes. Weil et al. [1975] have categorized and estimated the size of six social classes as follows: traditional elite (2%), new upper class (3%), middle class (15%), urban working class (semiskilled, 20%), urban lower class (minimum wage earners, 35%), and the marginal poor (25%).

Brazil's predominant ethnic group, estimated to be 60% of the population, is of European descent. The remaining 40% includes African (7%), Amerindian (1%), Japanese (less than 1%), and a large interracial group of European, African, and Amerindian [Weil et al., 1975].

Economically, Brazil is both an agricultural and an industrial country. Although industry is responsible for a large percentage of the gross national product (GNP), agriculture still plays an important role in the economy. In 1975, 45% of export earnings were provided by agricultural products including coffee, cattle, sugar, soybeans, cotton, and cocoa. Brazil ranks among the top five countries in the production of coffee, bananas, sisal, beans, manioc (cassava), sugar, soybeans, maize, oranges, cocoa, jute, beef, and tobacco [Dickenson, 1978].

Natural resources, such as timber, nuts, natural waxes, iron ore, gold, other metals and minerals, are abundant. Coal and petroleum resources (fossil fuels), however, are lacking. Alternate energy sources such as alcohol (made from cane sugar), hydroelectric power, and nuclear energy have been investigated to decrease reliance on petroleum imports.

Agriculture's role in Brazil's economy decreased as industrialization expanded. Industrialization progressed rapidly after the military coup in 1964. Described as an economic 'miracle', Brazil experienced GNP growth rates greater than 10% in the late 1960s to the early 1970s. These economic results were compatible with the government's developmental philosophy of rapid economic growth. Little attempt was made to decrease existing socioeconomic disparities. Government believed that economic and social benefits would eventually 'trickle down' to the population.

The economic boom, therefore, had relatively little positive economic and social impact for the majority of Brazilians. Although profits gained from the rapid growth of the industrial sector provided financial benefits for a small group of skilled laborers and the upper classes, the other social classes remained relatively unaffected [Nyrop, 1983]. One explanation was that the availability of a large labor force was ignored in the industrialization strategy. Industries, instead, used capital-intensive techniques.

Income distribution also remained highly skewed. The gap between the rich and the poor actually increased [Hewlett, 1980]. An estimated 40% of the country's income was acquired by the upper 5% of the population [Nyrop, 1983]. The lower 50% of the population received less than 12% of the country's total income [Nyrop, 1983]. The net result of Brazil's rapid economic growth was to widen the gap between the rich and the poor, and to increase regional disparity, with few positive economic and social benefits for most Brazilians [Hewlett, 1980].

Current international recession has had particularly detrimental effects on developing countries such as Brazil. Leading the Third World countries, Brazil has a foreign debt greater than 90 billion dollars, three digit inflation, massive unemployment, and crop failures due to regional floods and drought.

Rapid industrialization during the 1960s and 1970s also resulted in massive rural-urban migration, particularly in the southeastern region of Sao Paulo state [Anonymous, 1979]. The percentage of urban population in Brazil increased from 41% in 1940 to more than 55% in 1970 [Shrimpton, 1975; Dickenson, 1978; Hewlett, 1980].

Many factors are believed to be involved in the migration phenomenon. Examples include malnutrition, drought, desire to improve health, social and economic conditions, and the inability of the agricultural sector to absorb the increasing labor force and to provide well-paid and regular employment.

Inability of urban centers to cope with the influx of migrants has resulted in an increase in slums or squatter settlements. Frequently located on the periphery of the city, the slums are the most rapidly growing sectors of urban centers [Basta, 1977]. The result is overcrowding, substandard housing, unhygienic environment, infectious diseases, and malnutrition.

The nature and magnitude of malnutrition in Brazil has been documented in several studies. The 1974 to 1975 National Household Expenditure Survey (ENDEF) conducted in Brazil indicated widespread moderate and severe deficits in energy intake, and a significant degree of malnutrition in children [Knight and Moran, 1979]. Filho et al. [1981] reported regional differences in the prevalence of moderate and severe protein-energy malnutrition (PEM). Other investigations by Jansen et al. [1977], examined the nutritional quality of household diets as affected by income, urbanization, and region. Low income groups were reported to have low intakes of calories, protein, calcium, riboflavin, and thiamin.

Specific nutritional studies of agricultural migrant workers *(Boias-Frias)* have only been conducted recently. Investigations of agricultural migrants' diets in Sao Paulo state by Desai et al. [1980] revealed inadequate intakes of calories, calcium, iron, vitamin A, niacin, and ascorbic acid.

Resolution of the malnutrition problem is complex, due to its multifactorial etiology. Malnutrition can occur not only as a result of inadequate food intake, but due to other social, cultural, and biological factors affecting food intake and utilization. Any strategy(ies) selected to reduce or eliminate the malnutrition problem should consider a knowledge of the following factors: etiological factors in malnutrition, nutritionally vulnerable groups in the population, and the nature, degree, and magnitude of malnutrition in the population.

Use of nutrition education as a nutrition intervention strategy has been suggested by several investigators [Al-Isi et al., 1975; Church and Doughty, 1976; Ghosh et al., 1977; Tragler et al., 1981; Praun, 1982]. Application of nutrition education theory is based on the assumption that ignorance or lack of nutrition knowledge plays an important role in the etiology of malnutrition. Al-Isi et al. [1975] also state that nutrition education may be particularly valuable in the presence of poverty because people could be taught how to maximize benefits from a limited income.

Few nutrition education programs for agricultural migrant workers or low income groups in Brazil have been reported. Drummond [1975], using the methodology of the Brazilian educator Paulo Freire, conducted a nutrition education program in northeastern Brazil. Wright et al. [1982] used education as a means of introducing the use of soybeans in *favela* (slum) households in Sao Paulo state.

Little government action can be expected for low income groups living in *favelas* because of the government's developmental philosophy. Furthermore, no measures have been introduced by government to decrease socioeconomic disparities among various income groups. This situation has worsened because of the current international recession. Brazil's massive foreign debt, triple digit inflation, high unemployment, and recent crop failures have compounded the problems of low socioeconomic groups.

Considering Brazil's economic situation and political philosophy, no widespread social reforms to improve conditions for the less privileged in Brazilian society can be anticipated. Use of nutrition education, in these circumstances, could be the most appropriate intervention strategy. Nutrition education could stimulate an awareness of how people could make best possible use of limited resources and how they could assume more responsibility for their nutrition and health. As Al-Isi et al. [1975] have stated, nutrition education may be of particular value where poverty exists because people could be taught how to obtain maximum benefits from limited resources.

This study was designed to introduce a simple, informal nutrition education program to women (target group) living in Vila Diogo, a rural *favela* in Sao Paulo state. Design of the nutrition education program was based on results obtained from a nutritional needs assessment. Information was obtained from dietary intake assessments, infant feeding practices, dietary preferences, food intake frequencies and anthropometry.

Methods and Materials

Design of the Study

A nutritional needs assessment was conducted among Brazilian women and children less than 5 years of age from a low socioeconomic level. The target group in this study were female heads of households living in a *favela* (slum) on the periphery of Nuporanga, a rural settlement in Sao Paulo state, Brazil.

An appropriate nutrition education program for the target group was designed on the basis of information obtained from a nutritional needs assessment. The assessment was conducted among the target group and children under 5 years of age, using dietary assessment, nutrition knowledge, beliefs/attitudes questionnaires, and anthropometry.

Formative and summative evaluations of the nutrition education program were conducted, using appropriately selected criteria and comparing nutrition knowledge scores before and after the program.

Study Location

Nuporanga. The study was conducted in Nuporanga, a rural settlement located in northeastern Sao Paulo state and connected by highway with the cities of Ribeirao Preto and Sao Paulo, a distance of 80 and 400 km, respectively. Nuporanga, with an estimated population of 5,000, was situated in the heart of a rich farming region. Types of farms included cattle, coffee, poultry, sugar cane, cotton, rice and soybeans.

Nuporanga was one of the most picturesque and well-kept villages of the region. Houses reflected architecture of recent times coexisting with older homes constructed in the Portuguese style; brightly painted and accented with colorful tiles and houseplants. Approximately 100 low-cost houses were located on the outskirts of the village. Two *favelas,* Vila Nova, consisting of about 15 families and Vila Diogo, with more than 70 families, were situated on the periphery of Nuporanga.

Nuporanga had a variety of business and services. Local industries in the area included a chicken hatchery, abattoir, and a milk collection depot. Examples of small cottage industries were dress-making, basket weaving, broom-making, and metal work.

Health services available were an 18-bed hospital without surgical facilities, 2 doctors, several dentists, and 1 state Public Health Post. The Health Post offered immunizations, prenatal classes, and other infant-related services such as free milk distribution to infants in need.

Education facilities included a primary and secondary school, and a preschool operated on a fee basis. A second preschool or daycare-type center offered playground facilities, a small lunch, and bath to young children at no cost.

Types of recreational facilities and entertainment available were a public swimming pool, week-end soccer games, pinball arcade, and games in some of the bars. A private club offered limited game facilities and a monthly dance.

Because many residents did not have private telephones, public phones were located on the main street. A public address system announced funerals and deaths, as well as playing recorded music during the evening.

Walking was the most popular transportation mode within the village. Cars, trucks, and bicycles were common, with farmers frequently using horse or horse and cart.

Nuporanga's water supply was obtained from artesian wells, and piped into individual homes. Some homes used clay water filters as no centralized water treatment existed.

Water costs doubled and charges for other town services tripled in cost when the new mayor assumed office in February 1983.

Vila Diogo. Vila Diogo was located on the periphery of Nuporanga, approximately a 15-min walk from the village center. The *favela* was bordered on one side by a small coffee farm and a major road leading to a nearby city on the other side.

Houses were situated on both sides of an earthen street, with 20 and 56 houses on each side, respectively. At the beginning of the *favela,* houses were located in close proximity to each other, becoming more widely spaced towards the end of the *favela.*

All houses in Vila Diogo were personally owned. Houses were generally small, with 3.5 as the average number of rooms. Natural lighting and ventilation in houses were poor due to lack of windows. Windows in most homes were open with wooden shutters. Roofs were made of tiles, most walls were constructed from cement, and floors were either packed earth or concrete.

Electricity and piped-in water were obtained from Nuporanga sources. Of all households interviewed, 62% had electricity; 71.4% of households had piped-in water, with 25% obtaining water from *favela* wells.

In contrast to Nuporanga, the environment in Vila Diogo was unhygienic. Sanitation in Vila Diogo was poor, with open gutters used as a sewage disposal system. Furthermore, 82.2% of respondents used open gutters and yards for toilet facilities. A large percentage of respondents (61.4%) disposed of garbage openly on the street or yard. Another factor contributing to an unhygienic environment was that almost two thirds of households owned dogs, cats, birds, chickens, or hogs.

Most residents commuted to Nuporanga by walking, with only one or two men owning bicycles. Men and women working as agricultural laborers were transported to and from location by large trucks.

Study Population

Survey Procedure. The study population consisted of 76 families living in the *favela* of Vila Diogo. Factors considered in the selection of this population were that the *favela* was well-established, and situated on the periphery of a rural settlement.

Initial contact with Vila Diogo residents was made with the assistance of one of the local doctors. Research personnel were introduced to one of the oldest women residents, who subsequently acted as a liaison between the residents and research personnel.

All families living in Vila Diogo were visited on an individual basis by research personnel and local interviewers. Names and birthdates of individual family members were identified and recorded. Birthdates of residents, if unknown, were obtained from hospital records. The purpose of the study was explained and written or verbal consent was obtained from women (target group) who agreed to participate. Permission to involve children under the age of 5 years was obtained from the parents or guardian. Participants were assured to confidentiality of information and the freedom to withdraw from the study at any time.

Of the 76 families living in Vila Diogo, 71 female household heads were approached to participate in the study. The remaining 5 households consisted of female household heads who were mentally incompetent or households which were headed solely by males. Fifty-six women (78.9%) consented to participate in additional interviews, using questionnaires. During the study, 9 women, who originally had consented to participate, were no longer able to continue (n = 47). All women who consented to participate in the study were personally interviewed by local interviewers using the following questionnaires: Demographic/Socioeconomic/Food Habits/Health-Related Practices, 24-Hour Food Recall, Food Frequency, Food Preferences, Infant Feeding Practices, Nutrition Knowledge, and Nutrition Attitudes/Beliefs.

The 24-Hour Food Recall, Food Frequency and Food Preferences Questionnaires used in this study had been developed, pretested and administered in previous Brazilian agricultural migrant studies; the Demographic/Socioeconomic/Food Habits/Health-Related Practices Questionnaire, previously used in other agricultural migrant studies, was modified for the present study. Nutrition Knowledge and Nutrition Attitudes/Beliefs Questionnaires were developed for this study, translated into Portuguese, and pretested in Brazil. Questionnaires were administered by personal interview and conducted in Portuguese by two local teachers, who had been trained by research personnel. All interviews were supervised by the primary investigator who had a basic knowledge of the local language.

Demographic and Socioeconomic Information, Food- and Health-Related Practices. Seventy-six households were enumerated, with a total population of 352. Almost one quarter of all households (23.2%) were headed solely by women, compared to 7% for men.

Age distribution was highly skewed, with more than one half of the population (59.5%) 20 years of age or less, and few old people. Household size appeared large, with 47.3 and 7.9% of all households reporting more than 4 and 8 persons per household, respectively.

Other demographic and socioeconomic information is reported in table 1. Although literacy rate and education level among residents were low, a larger proportion of male household heads compared to females reported receiving formal education and being able to read and write. Years of formal education were low, with most residents not reporting more than 4 years. Furthermore, years of schooling reported may have included repeated grades. Reasons most frequently cited by mothers for children's poor school attendance records were that children disliked school (35.7%) and children were working, either because of personal preference or for economic reasons (28.6%).

For women who consented to participate in the study, a mean residency of 6.3 years in the present home was reported. Only a small percentage of respondents (14.2%) had migrated from other towns, states, or cities. A significant number of women (25%) were born and raised in Vila Diogo or had lived in another house in the same *favela;* 28.6 and 25% of respondents had previously lived in Nuporanga and *fazendas,* respectively. Reasons most frequently cited for moving to the Nuporanga district were to earn more money and to obtain better medical services.

Reported unemployment rates one week prior to interview were negligible, probably because agricultural work was nearing peak levels. Additional evidence, however, indicated that for women and children normally employed, significant numbers (18.2 and 10.8%, respectively) had different jobs between the time period of one month and one week prior to the survey.

The majority of households (62.5%) consisted of one wage earner supporting an average of 4.1 persons. As number of wage earners per household increased, mean number of household members generally increased.

Table 1. Demographic and socioeconomic characteristics of the study population[a]

	Household heads		Children
	male	female	
Ability to read and write	61.3	42.3	–
Formal education			
None	33.9	45.0	–
< 1–4 years	64.6	52.2	–
Children currently attending school	–	–	43.4
Employment rate[b]	97.5	100.0	97.3
Occupation[c]			
Agricultural laborer	70.0	72.7	62.2
Domestic	0	9.1	10.8
Other[d]	27.5	0	16.2
Estimated weekly income[e]			
Agricultural laborer	11.01–27.53	11.01–27.53	11.01–27.53
Domestic	–	–	3.28–4.59
Other[d]	5.24–27.53	–	–

[a] All values expressed as percent of total responses, unless otherwise noted.
[b] Employment rate one week prior to interview for persons normally employed.
[c] Type of employment one month prior to interview.
[d] Garbage collector, tractor operator, brick layer, making brooms, weeding gardens, mechanics' assistants, working in abattoir.
[e] Values expressed as US dollars.

Small cottage industries such as broom-making, basket weaving, shoe repairs, and soap-making for home use existed in the *favela.* The majority of men, women, and children who were employed, however, worked as agricultural laborers, with earnings varying widely, depending on the quantity of work performed (influenced by the individual's stamina, motivation, and health) as well as the weather. Wages for most occupations were below Brazilian minimum wage guidelines of $15.45 per week (US).

Recreational facilities in Vila Diogo were lacking, although men and boys used the street to play a game resembling horseshoes or a nearby field to play soccer. Men generally spent a good deal of leisure time in local village bars. Activities women most frequently reported when not working were visiting friends or family, sleeping, or resting. Young children played on the street with limited available toys.

Although voting is compulsory in Brazil, only about one third of women voted in the November 1982 elections for municipal, state, and federal representatives, compared to two thirds of men. Reasons most frequently given for not voting were the inability to read and write, and not having the necessary documents (i.e. identity card).

Dental health among *favela* residents was poor. Although free dental services were available, services were not used. *Favela* residents were also not charged for physician's services and women received free oral contraceptives. Local hospital and state Public Health Post services were frequently used. Approximately 95% of *favela* children, for example, were reported immunized against communicable diseases [personal communication]. Diseases such as malaria and Chaga's were no longer prevalent in the area. Common health problems reported for Vila Diogo children were respiratory infections and worm infestation, especially round worm and hookworm [personal communication].

A large percentage of men (75%) compared to women (44.6%) were reported smokers, with the majority smoking 10 cigarettes or less per day. Although some young children smoked, accurate information regarding children's smoking habits was difficult to obtain from mothers.

Alcohol consumption among men appeared excessive. Women generally reported a dislike of alcoholic beverages, although a few women reported consuming alcohol on an infrequent basis.

An investigation of women's reproductive history revealed a mean age of menstruation of 13.3 years (range 10–17 years), with mean age at first pregnancy (mean 20.2 years; range 14–37 years) occurring significantly later. The percentage of women reporting spontaneous abortions, stillbirths, and infant deaths was high (33.9, 10.7, and 25%, respectively), with a mean of 2.3 (range 1–8), 1.3 (range 1–2), and 1.5 (range 1–4), respectively.

At the time of the study, only 9% of women interviewed were pregnant or lactating. Of women who were not pregnant, a large percentage (46.4%) practised contraception, despite 84% of women indicating Roman Catholicism as their religion. Oral contraceptives were the most popular family planning method, accounting for 69.2% of all responses. Menopause, post menopausal age, living alone, and being widowed were reasons most frequently cited for women not practising contraception; religion was not a major factor. Mean birth interval, calculated for families with more than one child (less than 5 years old), was relatively large at 2.3 years.

In an attempt to determine desired family size, women were asked what family size they would currently consider appropriate for people like themselves. Almost one half of respondents indicated a similar family size to their own, with almost one third of respondents stating that a larger family size than their own would be recommended.

Regarding food-related practices, the majority of respondents (80.4%) reported growing some vegetables and/or having fruit trees on their property, with onion, chayote, manioc, okra, oranges, bananas, *limao,* and papaya as the most commonly grown vegetables and fruit. Food preservation was not generally practised, except for occasional drying of coffee beans.

Food supplies were almost totally purchased at Nuporanga supermarkets, usually on a once-a-week basis. Purchases were made almost equally by male and female household heads and transported to the homes by truck or van.

Meals were usually prepared by women using cooking facilities inside the house, with 80% of respondents using gas or a combination of gas and wood as cooking fuel. Although wood as cooking fuel was obtained at no charge, costs of cooking gas increased significantly, doubling in price during the study period.

More than one half of respondents (57.1 %), who had previously lived in other areas, reported changes in dietary patterns when moving to Vila Diogo. Milk was the most frequently mentioned food consumed by respondents at their former residence, but not in Vila Diogo because of the cost. Vegetables and meat (including organ meat) were foods currently consumed in Vila Diogo, but which had not been readily available and, therefore, not generally consumed at their former residence.

In summary, residents of Vila Diogo were a relatively well-established population living at or below poverty levels, and having a low literacy rate and education level. Furthermore, their physical environment was unhygienic and a contributing factor to health problems, especially among young children. Considering the described socioeconomic characteristics of Vila Diogo residents, nutritional problems, especially in young children, would be expected.

Vila Diogo women recognized their poor socioeconomic situation and were anxious to improve their property and financial condition. Supporting evidence was obtained from responses on how women would use money if they won the lottery. The majority of women indicated that houses would be improved or better houses constructed, and money would be deposited in the bank. Furthermore, almost one third (29.1 %) of women thought food intakes were inadequate and stated that they would purchase food in larger quantities. Only a small percentage of respondents (10.7 %) stated they would purchase empty energy foods such as sweets and carbonated beverages.

Although most respondents enjoyed living in Vila Diogo, several improvements for the *favela,* such as installation of a sewage system, an improved street, and piped-in water and electricity for all homes, were suggested.

Nutritional Assessment

Dietary Analyses. The 24-hour food intake of all children aged 2–5 years and women participating in the study was obtained by personal interview with the female head of the household, using a 24-Hour Food Recall Questionnaire. Quantities were expressed in Brazilian household measures: *colher de cha* (teaspoon), *colher de sopa* (soup spoon), *espumadeira* (slotted spoon), *concha* (ladle), *copo* (glass), *xicara de cha* (tea cup), *xicara de cafe* (coffee cup), *prato* (plate).

All 24-hour food intake interviews were conducted by one trained interviewer to maintain a degree of conformity in the interviewing procedure. Interviews were conducted during weekdays to determine intake during the week as well as Sunday, a day when food intake tended to vary.

Food preferences, frequency of food intake, and nutrition knowledge and attitudes and beliefs of women participating in the study were obtained by personal interview with the aid of the following questionnaires: Food Preferences, Food Frequency, Nutrition Knowledge, and Nutrition Attitudes/Beliefs.

Infant feeding practices of children under 2 years of age were determined by personal interview with the mother using the Infant Feeding Practices Questionnaire.

Anthropometric Measurements. Participants were invited to attend anthropometric measurement sessions which were conducted in one of the *favela* homes. Initial anthropometric measurements included height, weight, head circumference, triceps skinfold (TSF) thickness, and mid-upper-arm circumference (MUAC). Subsequent monthly height and weight measurements for children (under 5 years) participating in the study were obtained for a 3-month period, with results plotted individually on growth charts. One copy of the growth chart was given to hospital records; the second copy was given to the mother.

Anthropometric measurements were conducted by the primary investigator according to the methods described by Jelliffe [1966]. All measurements were obtained in the morning before the first main meal.

Weight. Subjects (women and children under 5 years) were weighed without shoes and wearing minimal clothing. No weight allowances were made for clothing. The balance, a single beam platform model, was calibrated prior to each weighing session. All weighings were read to the nearest 0.1 kg. Weights of infants and toddlers were determined by subtracting the weight of the mother from the total weight of the mother and infant.

Height. The height of all subjects greater than 100 cm was determined, using a telescopic vertical measuring rod attached to the single beam platform balance. Subjects were asked to remove shoes and stand erect with the back of the head touching the upright measuring rod and with the head held in the Frankfort plane. Measurements were recorded to the nearest 0.5 cm.

Crown-to-heel length of infants was determined by means of a recumbent length board, according to the method described by Jelliffe [1966]. Measurements were read to the nearest 0.1 cm.

Heights of children less than 100 cm were determined with the aid of the recumbent length board located in a vertical position. Measurements were read to the nearest 0.1 cm.

Head Circumference. Measurement of head circumference was determined for children 2 years of age or less. A flexible tape was placed firmly around the frontal bones, passing the tape around the head above the ears and over the maximal prominence at the back of the head [Jelliffe, 1966]. Measurements were read to the nearest 0.1 cm.

Mid-Upper-Arm Circumference. The MUAC of all subjects was determined with the aid of a flexible, plasticized tape. The tape was placed snugly around a freely hanging left arm at a point halfway between the acromion and olecranon. Measurements were read to the nearest 0.1 cm.

Triceps Skinfold Thickness. TSF thickness was measured in all subjects with the aid of a Lange caliper which exerted a constant pressure of 10 g/mm^2. The measurement was obtained with the left arm hanging in a relaxed position and at the site used for the measurement of the MUAC, as described by Jelliffe [1966]. An average of three individual readings was recorded to the nearest 0.1 mm.

Mid-Upper-Arm Muscle Circumference. Using values obtained for MUAC and TSF, the mid-upper-arm muscle circumference (MUAMC) was calculated according to the following formula [Jelliffe, 1966]:

$$\text{MUAMC} = \text{MUAC} - \pi \times \text{TSF}.$$

Anthropometric measurements were compared to national [Marcondes et al., 1968] and international [National Center for Health Statistics, NCHS, 1979] standards.

Nutrition Education Intervention Program

Development and Implementation. Results obtained from demographic and socioeconomic questionnaire and nutritional needs assessment confirmed that design and implementation of a nutrition education program was considered the most appropriate nutrition intervention strategy. Six topics selected for the nutrition education program were: Importance of Foods for Better Health, Measuring and Monitoring Growth and Nutrition of Children, Breast-Feeding, Feeding Young Children for Better Health, Nutrition of the Mother, and Socioeconomic Aspects about Food. Individual lessons were adapted from 'Guidelines for Training Community Health Workers in Nutrition' [WHO, 1981b] and 'Nutrition for Developing Countries' [King et al., 1972]. Although this nutrition education material had been prepared for use in developing countries, lessons had not been previously used nor pretested in Brazil.

Anticipated barriers to participation in the nutrition education program were lack of interest and motivation; weather (too hot, rain), or if weather was nice, potential participants could be working in the fields or visiting in the village; disruption of household routine, participants could think they were unable or too old to learn, some participants could be mentally incompetent; illness; participants could be cautious or suspicious; children could prevent some potential participants from attending; families and friends could be resentful or jealous; lack of energy and stamina; politics within the *favela.*

Possible motivating factors for participation in the nutrition education program could include curiosity, desire for social interaction, to have a change from the household environment, or desire to improve the family's welfare.

A group discussion with the two local interviewers, local doctor, and research personnel was held to determine duration of the nutrition education program, length of individual sessions, number of sessions per week, and location.

All women who had consented to participate in the study were approached on an individual basis and informed of the nutrition education program. Women were asked to state their preference for day of the week and time of day for the program. Three afternoons per week (Tuesdays, Thursdays, and Saturdays) were initially selected on the basis of the anticipated number of participants and the week days women considered most convenient.

Vila Diogo was selected as the site for the nutrition education program. Selection of Vila Diogo as opposed to a site in the village was based on the following considerations: temperature – if hot, women might be reluctant to walk to the village; distance; convenience for women with small children – children could be brought to the sessions; participant's familiarity with the environment.

Three women in Vila Diogo granted permission to use their yards or homes as sites for the nutrition education sessions. Criteria used to select locations included women's interest and enthusiasm in the study, physical size of the yard or home, and location of the site with respect to easy accessibility for most potential participants.

A 10-week time period was selected for conducting the nutrition education program, allowing 2 weeks for most nutrition topics. One hour, considered the maximum time for each session, was based on the high probability of a short attention span in women, hot weather, potential disruption by young children, and the need to minimize disruption of women's household routines. A snack at the conclusion of each session was planned to allow further social interaction and to provide an incentive for future attendance.

Factors considered in the presentation of the nutrition topics were: topics should be presented at a basic level of knowledge, topics should be presented in an informal manner with as many simple illustrations as possible, vocabulary used should be easily understood by the audience, concepts presented should be reinforced by repetition, and active participation from the audience should be encouraged by questioning participants and by informal discussion.

Two local interviewers were selected as instructors for the nutrition education program, based on the following factors: interviewers had pleasing personalities and had already established rapport with participants in the study, the interviewers were local village residents, interviewers had teaching experience, and one of the interviewers had a background in the health sciences.

Approximately one week prior to each nutrition education session, a meeting was held between instructors and research personnel. The content of each lesson was discussed, any questions answered, and suggestions for improving subsequent sessions were made.

One day prior to the first nutrition education session, instructors and primary investigator personally contacted all participants in the study and invited participants to attend. Subjects were informed of the number of nutrition education sessions per week, length of each session, and location.

Evaluation. Types of evaluation conducted were formative and summative, with formative evaluation used as a basis for improvements or changes in subsequent nutrition education sessions. Written evaluations by instructors and primary investigator were completed at the end of each nutrition education session using specified guidelines.

Summative evaluation, conducted on completion of the nutrition education program, consisted of written evaluations by instructors and primary investigator using suggested guidelines. In addition, program participants completed the Nutrition Knowledge Questionnaire to determine whether any changes in nutrition knowledge had occurred as a result of the education program.

Data Analyses

Computer programs, developed by Lewis James, formerly of the Faculty of Arts Computing Center, were used for nutrient analysis. Estimated daily nutrient intakes and percentage contribution of food groups to nutrient intake were determined for Vila Diogo women and children, age 2–5 years.

Wilcoxon signed rank test was used to determine whether differences in women's nutrition knowledge scores were statistically significant at $\alpha = 0.05$ and $\alpha = 0.01$.

Results

Results are presented in four categories: dietary assessment which includes infant feeding practices, women's food preferences and frequency of food intake, and 24-hour food intakes of women and children (2–5 years); anthropometric assessment of women and children (less than 5 years); nutrition knowledge, attitudes, and beliefs of women; and evaluation of the nutrition education program.

Nutritional Assessment

Dietary Assessment

Infant Feeding Practices. The age at which children (less than 5 years of age) were weaned is reported in table 2. Although all children had been breast-fed at birth, duration of breast-feeding was relatively short, with majority of infants no longer breast-feeding at 6 months of age. Sudden weaning was reported by numerous women (47.6%), with fewer women (38.2%) reporting gradual weaning practices. Women generally used a more expensive product such as powdered whole milk, rather than diluted cow's milk as a breast milk supplement or substitute.

The age at introduction of various liquids (other than milk), semi-solid and solid foods, reported in table 3, shows that tea (herb tea with sugar) and coffee (with sugar) were the most common beverages given to infants. By 6 months of age, most infants were consuming tea (herb tea with sugar) and about one half of infants were drinking coffee (with sugar). Fruit juices (with sugar) were popular and were generally introduced during 1–3 months of age. Although recommended infant feeding practices indicate milk alone is sufficient for infants up to 3–4 months of age, a small percentage of infants were given solids, such as bread, fruit, vegetables,

Table 2. Distribution of weaning age by children less than 5 years

Age groups	n	%	Cumulative, %
Up to 2 weeks[a]	3	15.8	15.8
2–3 weeks	1	5.3	21.1
1–3 months	8	42.0	63.1
4–6	2	10.5	73.6
7–9	3	15.8	89.4
10–12	1	5.3	94.7
1–1.5 years	1	5.3	100.0
	19	100.0	

[a] All infants were breast-fed at birth.

Table 3. Age at introduction of liquid, semi-solid, and solid foods (% of total responses)

	Months						
	<1	1–3	4–6	7–9	10–12	>13–<24	none[a]
Liquids/semi-solids							
Sugar water	0	38.1	0	0	0	0	61.9
Tea (herb tea with sugar)	23.8	42.8	14.3	4.8	0	0	14.3
Coffee (with sugar)	0	23.8	23.8	0	4.8	9.5	38.1
Soft drinks	0	4.8	14.4	4.8	4.8	4.8	66.4
Fruit juices (with sugar)	0	52.3	9.6	4.8	0	0	33.3
Gruel (cornstarch, manioc)	2.4	9.6	7.2	4.8	2.4	0	73.6
Soup (e.g. rice/bean)	0	19.0	28.7	4.8	4.8	0	42.7
Solids							
Bread	0	33.3	42.8	9.5	9.5	0	4.9
Fruit/vegetables	0	11.9	38.0	0	4.8	0	45.3
Rice	0	23.8	47.7	9.5	0	9.5	9.5
Beans	0	9.6	47.6	9.5	4.8	9.5	19.0
Eggs/meat/fish	0	19.0	26.2	9.5	7.2	2.4	35.7
Regular family food	0	4.8	28.4	19.2	23.8	9.6	14.2

[a] Responses included those infants who were not given the stated food item and infants who might not yet be at the age where the particular food item would be introduced.

Table 4. Infant feeding practices during illness

Feeding practices	Fever		Diarrhea		Other illnesses	
	n	%	n	%	n	%
Feed infants the same as when they are well	9	42.9	7	33.3	13	61.9
Do not give infants anything to eat or drink	0	0	4	19.1	1	4.8
Give infants only drinks	5	23.8	2	9.5	2	9.5
Give infants purges	–	–	8	38.1	0	0
Other	7[a]	33.3	0	0	5[b]	23.8
Total	21	100.0	21	100.0	21	100.0

[a] Includes: soup, tea and cookies, gruel made from wheat flour.
[b] Not known.

rice, beans, egg, meat, or regular family food early in life (1–3 months of age). Furthermore, by 6 months of age, one third of infants were already eating the regular adult diet.

Results of infant feeding practices during illness (table 4) found many practices to be nutritionally detrimental. Many infants were fed differently when ill, especially during fever and diarrhea. When infants had diarrhea, a large proportion were not given anything to eat nor drink, and were given laxatives; during fever, a large percentage of infants were only given liquids. Mothers, however, generally did not feed infants differently during other illnesses.

Food Preferences of Women. Female heads of households (n = 47) were asked to state their degree of preference of numerous food items. The most popular food item for each degree of preference is recorded in table 5.

A unanimous preference was noted for many vegetables, including the yellow and dark green types. Egg plant, which was commonly available, was disliked by a significant percentage of respondents. Beans (legume group) and rice (cereal group) were highly preferred, which is explained by the cultural basis of rice and beans in Brazilian diets. Regarding dairy products, cheese, not milk, was the food item preferred by most respondents. Chicken and liver were preferred by all women. In the fruit group, only *jaboticaba* was unanimously preferred by all respondents. Beverages preferred by most women were coffee with sugar (Brazil's national beverage), *guarana* (a carbonated Brazilian drink), and chocolate. Although soybeans were disliked by a significant percentage of women, soybean oil was preferred by most women.

Women generally expressed preferences for a variety of food, although a significant number of respondents indicated a dislike of readily available products such as soybeans and egg plants.

Frequency of Food Intake by Women. Female household heads (n = 47) were asked to indicate frequency of consumption of specified food items. The most popular foods consumed are reported in table 6. Although the majority of women had previously reported preference for a wide variety of foods, daily food intake in terms of variety was very limited. Foods generally consumed on a daily basis were rice, beans, and coffee with sugar. Chicken, liver, and cheese, although highly preferred, were infrequently consumed. Vegetable intake was generally low, with onions used once a day and chayote several times per week. Intake of fruit and empty energy

Table 5. Foods most frequently preferred by female household heads[a]

Food group	Like	Dislike	Never tried/unfamiliar
Dairy products	cheese (96)	goat milk (23)	goat milk (53)
Meat/eggs	chicken (100)	shrimp (28)	cat (89) goat (62) mutton (62)
Organ meats	liver (100)	brain (28)	brain (11)
Legumes	beans (98) (excluding soybeans)	soybeans (38)	lentils (64)
Cereals	rice (100) bread rolls (100) wheat flour (100)	oatmeal (28)	whole wheat bread (51)
Vegetables	manioc[b] (100) corn (100) tomato (100) chayote (100) onion greens (100) wild chicory (100)	egg plant (55)	manioc[b] leaves (79)
Fruits	*jaboticaba*[c] (100)	*jatoba*[d] (58)	nectarine (89)
Beverages	coffee with sugar (94) *guarana*[e] (94) chocolate (94)	coffee without sugar (74)	*pinga*[f] (40)
Sweets/desserts	unrefined sugar (100)	honey (15)	refined sugar (2) cakes/biscuits (2)
Nuts/seeds	coconut (79)	cashew nut (30) cotton seed (30)	jak fruit seed (57) cotton seed (57)
Fats/oils	margarine (96) soybean oil (96)	beef fat (43)	cocoa butter (53)
Condiments	tomato sauce (100) salt (100)	ginger (13) bay leaf (13) red pepper (13)	paprika (83)

[a] Figures in parentheses express percent of respondents.
[b] Cassava.
[c] Round dark red-purple fruit the size of a cherry.
[d] A tropical fruit.
[e] Carbonated drink made from a small red Amazonian berry (guarana).
[f] A crude rum made from sugar cane.

Table 6. Frequency of food consumption by female household heads[a]

Food group	Daily	2–3 times per week	Once in a while	Never
Dairy products	powdered milk (11)	skim milk (4)	cheese (70)	goat milk (96)
Meat/eggs	eggs (17)	beef (21)	chicken (85)	cat (100) goat (98)
Organ meats	0	liver (2)	liver (79)	brain (49)
Legumes	beans (91) (excluding soybeans)	beans (2)	dried peas (34)	lentils (91) soybeans (91)
Cereals	rice (100)	macaroni (28)	macaroni (55)	arrowroot (94)
Vegetables	onion (64)	chayote (23)	potato (87) manioc[b] (87)	manioc[b] leaves (96) beet leaves (96)
Fruits	*limao*[c] (28)	banana (9)	avocado (83) banana (83) Brazilian tangerine (83)	nectarine (98) grapefruit (89)
Beverages	coffee with sugar (91)	*guarana*[d] (6)	carbonated beverages (72)	*pinga*[e] (98)
Sweets/desserts	unrefined sugar (96)	ice cream (2) unrefined sugar (2) cakes/biscuits (2)	ice cream (68)	refined sugar (79)
Nuts/seeds	0	0	peanuts (45)	jak fruit seeds (94) cashew nuts (94)
Fats/oils	butter (15) margarine (15)	butter (2) pork fat (2) olive oil (2)	soybean oil (85)	cocoa butter (94)
Condiments	salt (100)	tomato sauce (4) pepper sauce (4)	tomato sauce (72)	paprika (98)

[a] Figures in parentheses express percent of respondents.
[b] Cassava.
[c] A fruit resembling a cross between a lemon and an orange.
[d] Carbonated drink made from a small red Amazonian berry (guarana).
[e] A crude rum made from sugar cane.

foods such as carbonated beverages occurred on an infrequent basis. From the limited number and variety of food intakes reported, most women would be expected to be at high risk for inadequate nutrient intake such as ascorbic acid, iron, calcium, riboflavin, and vitamin A.

Most respondents (85.7%) reported that dietary patterns varied on certain days of the week or special occasions, especially Sundays and

Christmas. Food or beverages most frequently consumed during these days or special occasions were macaroni, chicken, other meat, wine, beer, or carbonated drinks. The reason most often cited by respondents (41.1 %) for eating these foods, particularly during these times, was that the family could not afford to buy these foods every day. Insufficient income is, therefore, probably a major factor in the difference observed between women's reported food preferences and frequency of food consumption.

24-Hour Food Intake. Women. The results of estimated mean daily nutrient intakes of Vila Diogo women (n = 37) and comparison with international standards are reported in table 7. Nutrients showing the greatest variation in intake, as indicated by the standard deviation, were vitamin A, riboflavin, and ascorbic acid, implying that a few women may have consumed foods rich in these nutrients.

Table 7. Comparison of estimated mean daily nutrient intakes of women with international standards[a]

Nutrient		Recommended daily intake	Mean intake ± SD	Daily intake < 2/3 FAO standard		Daily intake < 1/3 FAO standard	
				n	%	n	%
Energy	kcal	2,200	1,426 ± 702.6	24	64.9	5	13.5
	MJ	9.2	5.99				
Protein, g		41[b]	41.7 ± 30.4	12	32.4	2	5.4
Calcium, mg		400	204.2 ± 176.1	30	81.1	17	45.9
Iron, mg		19[c]	7.17 ± 3.76	33	89.2	17	45.9
Vitamin A, RE		750	2,685.9 ± 673.2	33	89.2	27	73.0
Thiamin, mg		0.9	0.62 ± 0.37	21	56.8	5	13.5
Riboflavin, mg		1.3	0.60 ± 0.90	33	89.2	16	43.2
Niacin, mg		14.5	7.63 ± 5.19	26	70.3	14	37.8
Ascorbic acid, mg		30	13.5 ± 23.7	32	86.5	25	67.6
α-Tocopherol, mg[d]		6[e]	5.53 ± 2.81	10	27.0	2	5.4

[a] Food and Agriculture Organization (FAO) [Beaton and Patwardhan, 1976].
[b] Based on mixed cereal-legume diet with small amounts of animal source foods.
[c] If proportion of energy derived from animal sources or soybean is 10–25 %.
[d] Based on α-tocopherol equivalents.
[e] Based on Canadian Recommended Daily Nutrient Intakes, 1983.

The Food and Agriculture Organization (FAO) standards with cut-off points of two thirds and one third of recommended levels were used to compare women's intakes. Brazilian standards were not available. Nutrients in which women most frequently failed to meet two thirds of FAO recommended levels were calcium, iron, vitamin A, riboflavin, and ascorbic acid. If women who did not meet one third of FAO levels for these nutrients continued these low intakes, they would probably be at a high risk for nutrient deficiencies. Protein and α-tocopherol were the nutrients in which women were most successful in achieving FAO recommended intakes.

The percentage contribution of food groups to women's nutrient intake, reported in table 8, indicated that cereals and legumes (specifically rice and beans) were the main sources of energy, protein, and calcium. Dairy products, a rich source of calcium, provided only a small percentage of calcium intake. Iron intake was obtained primarily from less readily absorbable nonheme sources such as legumes. Vitamin-A-rich foods (animal protein, dairy products, dark yellow and green vegetables) provided only a small proportion of total vitamin A intake; legumes accounted for the majority of vitamin A intake. Thiamin, riboflavin, and niacin intakes were provided mainly by legume and animal protein sources, with negligible amounts contributed by dairy sources. The majority of ascorbic acid intake originated from vegetables (other than dark green and yellow types) rather than fruit.

The percentage contribution of various food groups to nutrient intake provided additional evidence that some women could be at high risk for inadequate intake of specific nutrients. Good sources of calcium (dairy products), ascorbic acid (fruit, dark green and yellow vegetables), vitamin A (meat, dairy products, dark green and yellow vegetables), iron (animal protein), and riboflavin (dairy products) provided little of the total daily intake. With a daily diet consisting primarily of rice, beans, and sweetened coffee, it is highly probable that this diet, lacking in variety, cannot adequately provide sufficient intakes of most nutrients, with the exception of α-tocopherol and protein.

The distribution of women's energy intake from macro-nutrients (table 9), however, was probably satisfactory. Almost one half of the total daily energy intake originated from complex carbohydrates, with only a small proportion being derived from simple sugars (sugar and carbonated beverages). Alcoholic beverages did not contribute to energy intake. Furthermore, diets were high in polyunsaturated fatty acids (e.g. linoleic acid) and relatively low in saturated fatty acids.

Table 8. Percentage contribution of food groups to nutrient intake of women

Nutrient		Dairy products	Animal protein sources	Food groups						
				vegetables				fruit	cereals	fats/oils
				legumes	dark green	dark yellow	other			
Energy	mean ± SD	1.3 ± 3.1	12.2 ± 13.7	26.3 ± 12.4	0.04 ± 0.1	0.2 ± 0.5	1.5 ± 2.7	0.5 ± 1.9	48.4 ± 12.0	4.7 ± 4.6
	range	0–11.6	0–44.3	0–47.0	0–0.7	0–1.9	0–14.5	0–8.6	22.2–69.1	0–14.6
Protein	mean ± SD	2.7 ± 5.8	31.0 ± 29.8	33.3 ± 19.6	0.2 ± 0.7	0.4 ± 1.0	1.4 ± 2.3	0.4 ± 1.8	30.6 ± 13.5	0
	range	0–20.2	0–91.7	0–62.9	0–3.5	0–3.5	0–6.3	0–9.7	8.3–55.7	0
Calcium	mean ± SD	12.7 ± 26.5	13.0 ± 19.1	28.1 ± 16.4	1.3 ± 4.7	1.2 ± 3.1	5.8 ± 10.7	2.2 ± 9.0	31.7 ± 13.8	0
	range	0–89.1	0–68.4	0–55.8	0–23.3	0–12.8	0–53.6	0–39.6	4.7–57.4	0
Iron	mean ± SD	1.1 ± 2.7	19.1 ± 21.2	54.2 ± 21.9	0.6 ± 2.2	0.7 ± 1.6	3.8 ± 5.5	1.2 ± 4.7	17.0 ± 7.2	0
	range	0–12.6	0–80.8	0–84.1	0–9.9	0–5.6	0–26.5	0–22.8	5.8–43.6	0
Vitamin A	mean ± SD	5.4 ± 13.5	17.4 ± 28.0	30.7 ± 30.7	5.0 ± 18.9	14.4 ± 33.2	13.7 ± 23.0	1.6 ± 6.8	1.5 ± 6.1	10.6 ± 12.6
	range	0–48.9	0–99.2	0–100.0	0–92.6	0–94.7	0–73.1	0–36.4	0–33.2	0–46.8
Thiamin	mean ± SD	1.5 ± 3.8	22.8 ± 24.9	48.8 ± 23.1	0.3 ± 0.9	0.7 ± 1.6	3.1 ± 4.2	1.8 ± 7.3	19.4 ± 9.6	0
	range	0–14.7	0–77.7	0–79.9	0–4.8	0–5.7	0–15.7	0–34.7	4.6–47.1	0
Riboflavin	mean ± SD	6.2 ± 13.8	34.8 ± 32.0	32.1 ± 22.4	0.8 ± 3.1	1.5 ± 3.8	5.7 ± 9.9	1.3 ± 5.3	14.2 ± 7.2	0
	range	0–52.4	0–95.0	0–74.0	0–17.9	0–15.2	0–44.5	0–24.9	1.9–28.3	0
Niacin	mean ± SD	0.3 ± 0.6	29.6 ± 30.8	19.3 ± 11.8	0.2 ± 0.7	0.7 ± 1.7	3.5 ± 5.8	0.5 ± 2.3	33.0 ± 16.2	0
	range	0–20.0	0–90.8	0–40.5	0–3.9	0–6.0	0–26.2	0–11.2	5.6–67.9	0
Ascorbic acid	mean ± SD	12.0 ± 30.8	2.8 ± 15.8	0	4.1 ± 17.9	13.2 ± 30.2	59.0 ± 46.2	9.0 ± 28.4	0	0
	range	0–100.0	0–89.1	0	0–100.0	0–100.0	0–100.0	0–100.0	0	0
α-Tocopherol	mean ± SD	0.5 ± 1.4	6.9 ± 11.3	38.8 ± 16.4	0.9 ± 3.7	0.8 ± 2.0	2.4 ± 4.7	0.1 ± 0.5	35.6 ± 11.8	13.3 ± 14.2
	range	0–5.9	0–33.0	0–60.8	0–20.5	0–7.0	0–25.5	0–2.4	1.7–63.2	0–61.5

Percentages of various food groups do not equal 100% because of rounding off of percentages and omission of miscellaneous items (e.g. sugar, coffee).

Table 9. Distribution of energy intake from macro-nutrients

Source	24-Hour energy distribution			
	women		children	
	kcal (MJ)	% of total energy	kcal (MJ)	% of total energy
Protein (total)	166.8 (0.70)	11.8	120.4 (0.51)	12.3
Carbohydrate (total)	700.8 (2.94)	49.1	464.4 (1.95)	47.4
Sugar	66.0 (0.28)	4.6	54.3 (0.23)	5.6
Carbonated drinks	6.1 (0.03)	0.4	30.6 (0.13)	3.2
Fat (total)	557.1 (2.34)	39.1	394.2 (1.67)	40.3
Saturated fatty acids	122.4 (0.51)	8.6	115.2 (0.48)	11.9
Oleic acid	160.2 (0.67)	11.2	123.3 (0.52)	12.7
Linoleic acid	232.2 (0.98)	16.3	124.2 (0.52)	12.8

No alcohol consumption was reported during the survey period.

Children. Daily nutrient intake of Vila Diogo children (n = 8) age 2–5 years was estimated by interviewing mothers using the 24-hour food recall method. Of all households who consented to participate, only 8 children were in the 2 to 5 year age group. Results of estimated mean daily intakes and comparison with FAO recommendations are reported in table 10.

Children's estimated daily nutrient intakes appeared more satisfactory than that reported by women. Although one half or more of children did not meet two thirds of FAO recommended levels for vitamin A, niacin, ascorbic acid, calcium, iron, and α-tocopherol, ascorbic acid was the only nutrient that one half of children were unsuccessful in meeting one third of FAO recommended intakes. Some children could, therefore, be at a high risk of ascorbic acid deficiency.

The percentage contribution of food groups to children's nutrient intake (table 11) indicated that energy intake was provided primarily by cereal sources (i.e. rice). Due to significant milk consumption, protein sources were almost equally derived from dairy products, animal protein, and cereals. Furthermore, dairy products were the main contributor of calcium and vitamin A intake. Some iron intake was obtained from more

Table 10. Comparison of estimated mean daily nutrient intakes of children with international standards[a]

Nutrient	Recommended daily intake	Mean intake ± SD	Daily intake < 2/3 FAO standard		Daily intake < 1/3 FAO standard	
			n	%	n	%
Energy kcal	1,360	971.7 ± 358.2	3	37.5	0	0
MJ	5.7	4.08				
Protein, g	23[b]	30.1 ± 13.7	1	12.5	0	0
Calcium, mg	400	359.3 ± 305.9	4	50.0	1	12.5
Iron, mg	7[c]	4.86 ± 2.23	4	75.0	1	12.5
Vitamin A, RE	250	1,184.9 ± 2,209.6	6	75.0	2	25.0
Thiamin, mg	0.5	0.53 ± 0.41	1	12.5	1	12.5
Riboflavin, mg	0.8	0.87 ± 1.10	3	37.5	1	12.5
Niacin, mg	9.0	5.02 ± 3.06	6	75.0	1	12.5
Ascorbic acid, mg	20	8.1 ± 5.9	7	87.5	4	50.0
α-Tocopherol, mg[d]	4[e]	2.98 ± 1.33	4	50.0	0	0

[a] Food and Agriculture Organization (FAO) [Beaton and Patwardhan, 1976].
[b] Based on mixed cereal-legume diet with small amounts of animal source foods.
[c] If proportion of energy derived from animal sources or soybean is 10–25%.
[d] Based on α-tocopherol equivalents.
[e] Based on Canadian Recommended Daily Nutrient Intakes, 1983.

readily absorbable heme sources (animal protein), with most iron intake, however, originating from less readily absorbable sources such as legumes and cereals. As was observed in women's nutrient intakes, no ascorbic acid was obtained from rich ascorbic acid sources such as fruit or dark green and yellow vegetables. Dairy products and animal protein, good sources of riboflavin, niacin, and thiamin, however, were the primary contributors to children's intakes of these nutrients. Distribution of children's energy intake from macro-nutrients was satisfactory and was similar to that reported for women (table 9).

Compared to women, children's nutrient intakes appeared more satisfactory, an observation probably explained by the high prevalence of milk consumption. Children's intake of ascorbic acid, however, was similar to that reported for women, and children could be at high risk, therefore, of ascorbic acid deficiency.

Table 11. Percentage contribution of food groups to nutrient intake of children

Nutrient		Dairy products	Animal protein sources	Food groups[a]				
				vegetables			cereals	fats/oils
				legumes	dark green	other		
Energy	mean ± SD	12.3 ± 13.8	16.1 ± 18.0	15.2 ± 5.5	0	1.5 ± 1.6	43.0 ± 17.2	5.4 ± 5.1
	range	1.7 – 39.9	0 – 57.4	3.1 – 19.6	0	0 – 3.9	20.5 – 71.2	0 – 13.8
Protein	mean ± SD	22.8 ± 19.2	28.1 ± 26.1	16.9 ± 8.5	0.2 ± 0.5	1.6 ± 1.7	30.4 ± 17.3	0
	range	3.2 – 52.5	0 – 71.2	1.8 – 30.8	0 – 1.2	0 – 4.2	7.7 – 60.3	0
Calcium	mean ± SD	66.0 ± 23.1	3.9 ± 6.0	8.5 ± 5.8	2.1 ± 4.3	2.5 ± 3.7	14.8 ± 11.3	0
	range	34.9 – 94.5	0 – 16.3	0.3 – 17.0	0 – 12.0	0 – 10.2	1.6 – 35.5	0
Iron	mean ± SD	10.8 ± 9.6	23.5 ± 23.6	36.3 ± 15.9	0.9 ± 2.1	4.3 ± 4.6	21.6 ± 8.7	0
	range	1.6 – 27.7	0 – 68.5	3.8 – 58.2	0 – 5.9	0 – 13.3	5.0 – 33.3	0
Vitamin A	mean ± SD	30.5 ± 26.6	18.5 ± 35.7	16.3 ± 18.5	12.7 ± 31.1	13.4 ± 15.7	0.4 ± 1.0	8.1 ± 7.7
	range	2.2 – 78.0	0 – 97.8	0 – 58.9	0 – 89.0	0 – 45.3	0 – 2.8	0 – 16.7
Thiamin	mean ± SD	16.6 ± 17.0	32.5 ± 22.8	27.6 ± 5.4	0.5 ± 1.0	4.1 ± 4.0	18.3 ± 11.0	0
	range	1.1 – 48.5	0 – 74.3	4.4 – 52.9	0 – 2.8	0 – 9.9	7.3 – 41.0	0
Riboflavin	mean ± SD	45.3 ± 25.1	30.2 ± 28.7	10.1 ± 6.9	0.6 ± 1.2	2.7 ± 3.2	9.2 ± 7.1	0
	range	11.9 – 86.7	0 – 69.8	0.3 – 24.4	0 – 2.8	0 – 9.0	0.6 – 24.4	0
Niacin	mean ± SD	4.1 ± 4.2	39.2 ± 33.5	17.9 ± 16.6	0.2 ± 0.4	15.7 ± 29.8	34.9 ± 22.4	0
	range	0.3 – 13.2	0 – 85.8	0.9 – 20.1	0 – 1.1	0 – 15.6	7.1 – 75.7	0
Ascorbic acid	mean ± SD	29.6 ± 32.4	8.6 ± 24.4	0	13.4 ± 32.6	45.9 ± 40.0	0	0
	range	2.8 – 100.0	0 – 68.9	0	0 – 93.3	0 – 89.4	0	0
α-Tocopherol	mean ± SD	4.3 ± 5.3	10.1 ± 18.6	30.2 ± 12.5	2.9 ± 7.9	1.9 ± 2.3	32.4 ± 17.1	18.0 ± 16.7
	range	0.7 – 14.4	0 – 54.5	6.6 – 45.3	0 – 22.5	0 – 6.3	20.3 – 65.2	0 – 43.9

[a] No intake was reported for fruit nor dark yellow vegetables.

Percentages of various food groups do not equal 100% because of rounding off of percentages and omission of miscellaneous items (e.g. sugar, coffee).

Anthropometric Assessment

Anthropometric Status of Women. The mean and range of several anthropometric measurements – weight, height, MUAC, TSF thickness, MUAMC – of women (table 12) indicated a wide range of values for weight and TSF thickness. Because local Brazilian standards were not available,

Table 12. Anthropometric measurements of women

	n	Mean ± SD	Range
Weight, kg	40	58.5 ± 14.5	36.7–93.5
Height, cm	40	150.2 ± 6.9	137.5–164.5
MUAC, cm	67	27.2 ± 4.1	18.6–37.4
TSF, mm	67	15.5 ± 6.2	4.0–29.0
MUAMC, cm	67	22.3 ± 2.8	17.3–28.7

Table 13. Comparison of women's anthropometric measurements with international standards[a]

	NCHS[b] percentiles							
	< 5	5	10	25	50	75	> 90	Total
Weight for height	8	1	6	5	6	4	2	32
% of total responses	25.0	3.0	18.8	15.6	18.8	12.5	6.3	100

	Frisancho percentiles[c]						
	< 5	5	15	50	85	> 95	Total
MUAC	3	2	10	14	8	3	40
% of total responses	7.5	5.0	25.0	35.0	20.0	7.5	100
TSF thickness	4	4	12	18	2	0	40
% of total responses	10.0	10.0	30.0	45.0	5.0	0	100
MUAMC	0	0	6	16	13	5	40
% of total responses	0	0	15.0	40.0	32.5	12.5	100

[a] Figures express number of responses.

[b] National Centre for Health Statistics.

[c] Frisancho [1974] – standards derived from Ten State Nutrition Survey (TSNS) data, 1968–1970.

anthropometric measurements were compared to the National Center for Health Statistics (NCHS) standards and Frisancho's standards (table 13). NCHS standards were derived from USA (HANES) data. The only standards available for MUAC, TSF, and MUAMC were prepared by Frisancho [1974] from Ten State Nutrition Survey (TSNS) data.

Results indicated that more than one half of women (62.4%) had weight-for-height values below the 50th percentile or median, implying that some women were probably underweight. A more significant observation was that 28% of women had weight-for-height values at or below the 5th percentile, indicating that a significant proportion of women were undernourished. Comparison of MUAC, TSF thickness, and MUAMC with Frisancho's standards confirmed that some women were exhibiting varying degrees of malnutrition. A large percentage of women (20%), for example, had TSF thickness at or below the 5th percentile, indicating that little or no energy reserves were present as fat.

Anthropometric Status of Children. Weight for Age. Weight for age was plotted graphically for children under the age of 5 years, using NCHS Growth Charts (fig. 2). Weights of children were compared to the 5th, 50th, and 95th NCHS percentiles and the Marcondes' 50th percentile. Marcondes' standards were derived from data obtained primarily from Brazilian low socioeconomic groups. As expected, lower anthropometric values, as noted by comparison of Marcondes' 50th percentile with NCHS values, were observed.

For the majority of boys (76.9%), weights for age were below NCHS's median (50th percentile), implying that a significant number of boys were underweight for their age. In contrast, fewer girls (65%) had weights less than the NCHS median.

Although weight for age results indicated some children were underweight, weight for age index does not consider children who, because of a small frame size, may have normal weights. The percentage of children who may be actually classified as underweight will be less than indicated by the weight for age index.

Height for Age. When height or length for age of children was compared to NCHS and Marcondes' standards (fig. 3), almost one half of boys (46.2%) and one third or girls (31.6%) had height-for-age values less than the NCHS 5th percentile. Because height for age is an indicator of past nutritional state, these results indicated that stunting appeared to exist in a

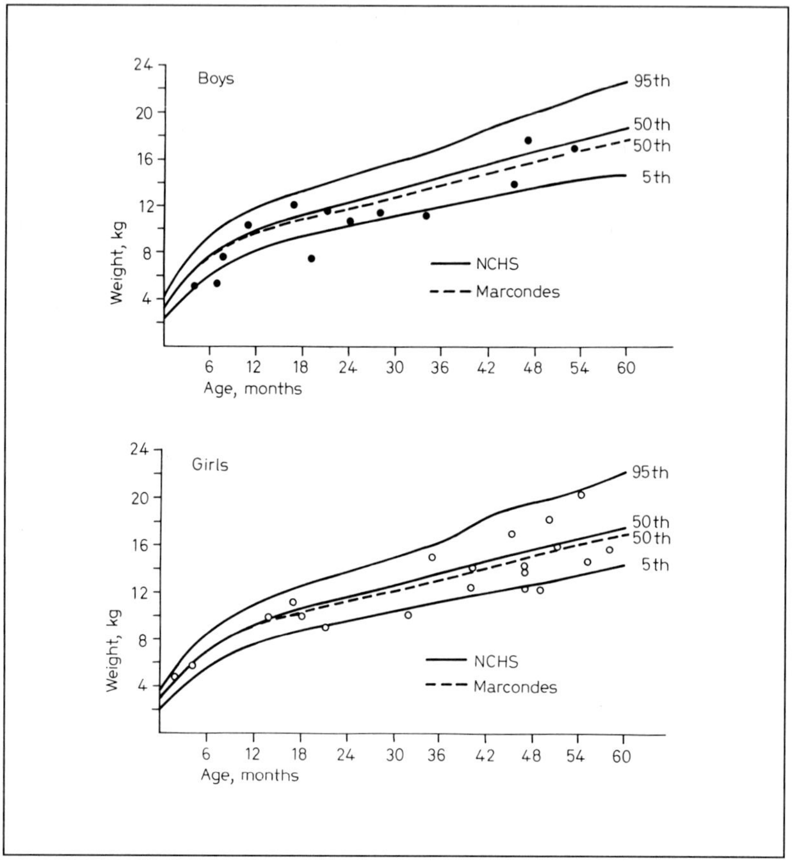

Fig. 2. Comparison of boys' and girls' weights for age with NCHS and Marcondes' percentiles.

significant percentage of children. Poor nutrition, therefore, was a likely factor involved directly or indirectly in stunted growth.

Weight for Height. Since weight-for-height or weight-for-length indices consider weight of subjects in terms of body frame size, subjects with a small frame but normal weight will not be classified as underweight or malnourished. The weight-for-height index, therefore, is a more accurate index than weight for age in describing the current nutritional state of children.

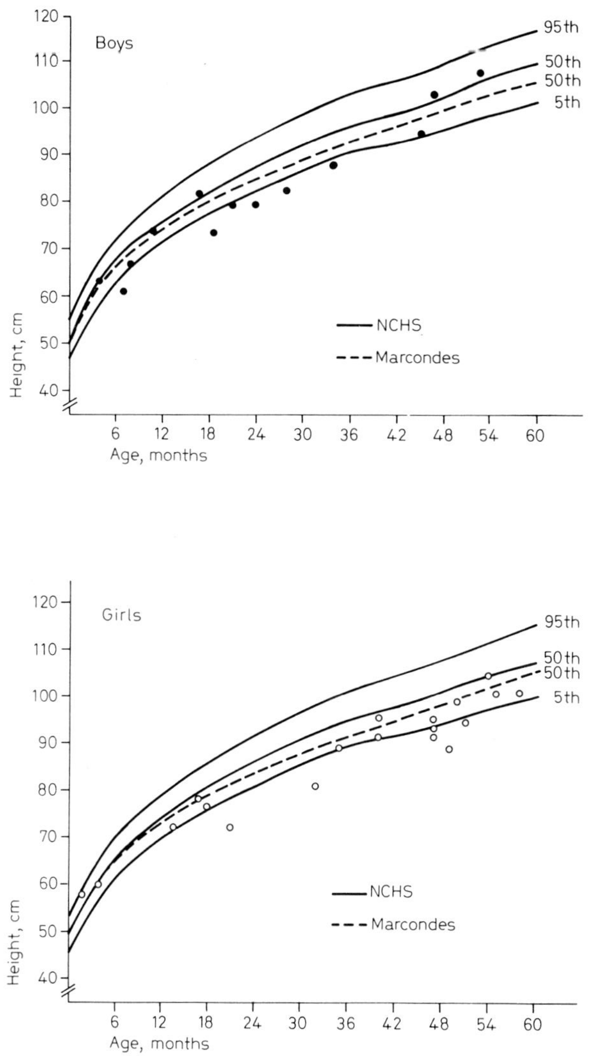

Fig. 3. Comparison of boys' and girls' height for age with NCHS and Marcondes' percentiles.

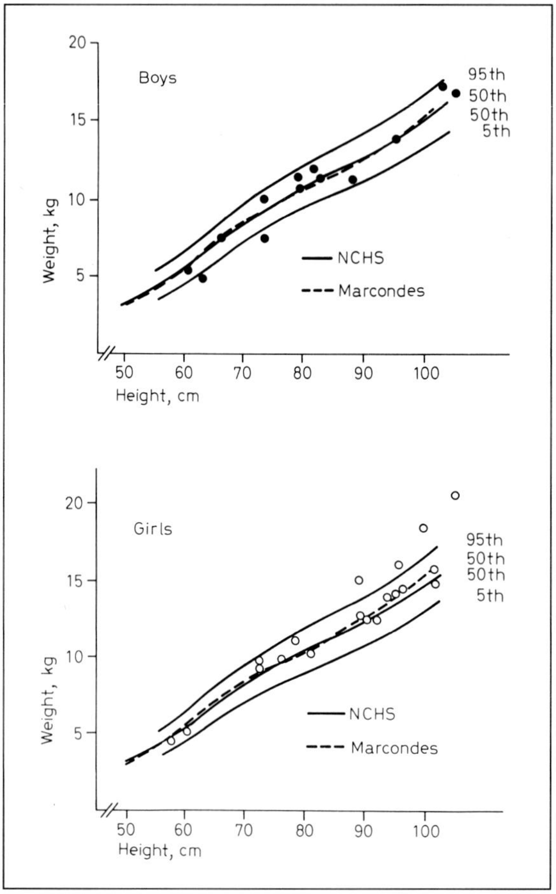

Fig. 4. Comparison of boys' and girls' weight for height with NCHS and Marcondes' percentiles.

A comparison of weight for height for children in this study with NCHS and Marcondes' percentiles (fig. 4) confirmed that fewer boys and girls had weight-for-height values below the NCHS 5th percentile compared to weight for age. Furthermore, the number of values below the NCHS median was about 50% less when the weight-for-height index was used compared to weight for age. Although many children were stunted in growth, the majority of children appeared to have satisfactory weights for body size.

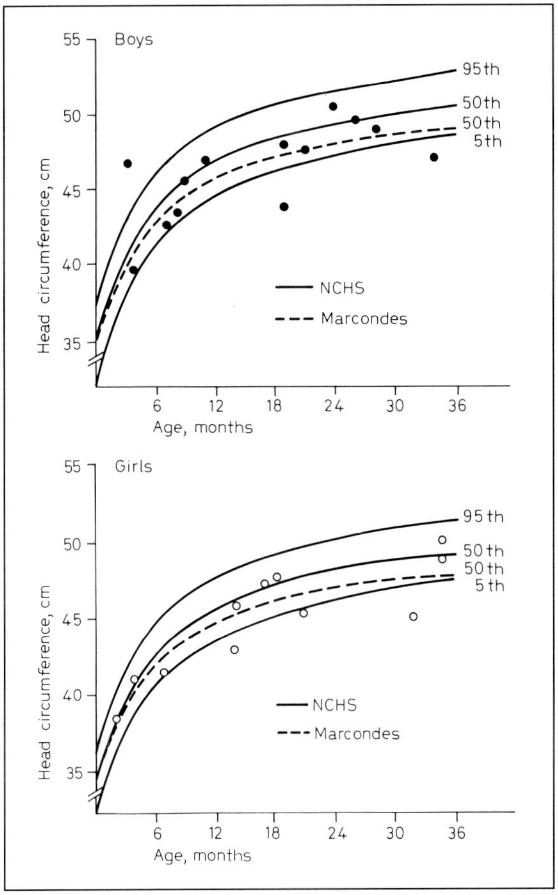

Fig. 5. Comparison of boys' and girls' head circumference for age with NCHS and Marcondes' percentiles.

Head Circumference. Head growth occurs most rapidly during the first few years of life. Use of head circumference (HC) measurements in children, therefore, is a sensitive indicator to measure the presence of current malnutrition.

HC of children less than 3 years of age was compared with NCHS and Marcondes' standards (fig. 5). Differences were observed between Marcondes' and NCHS's 50th percentiles. Although difficulties in conducting measurements could perhaps partially explain some of the extreme values

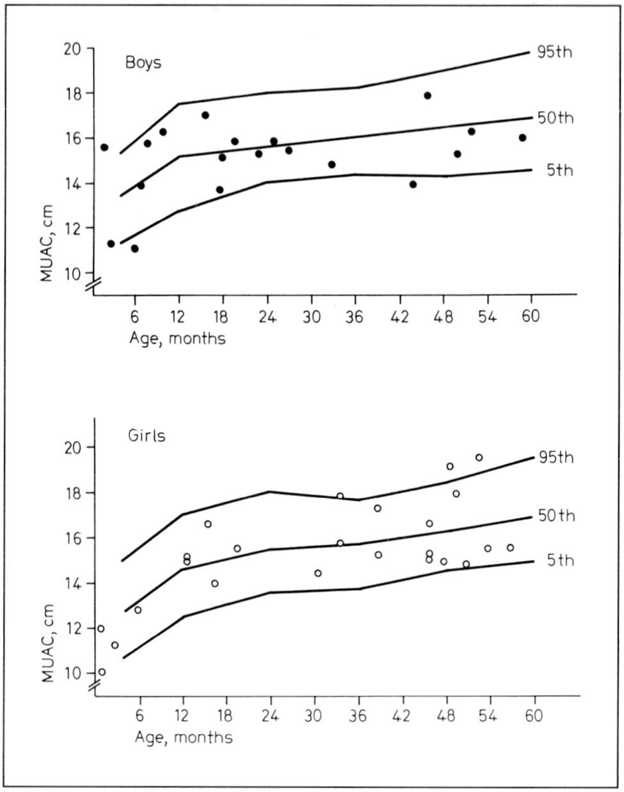

Fig. 6. Comparison of boys' and girls' MUAC with TSNS percentiles.

obtained, more boys than girls (61.5 vs. 45.5%) had values below the NCHS 50th percentile. Some young children were, therefore, probably not growing adequately due to poor nutrition.

Mid-Upper-Arm Circumference, Triceps Skinfold Thickness, and Mid-Upper-Arm Muscle Circumference. The MUAC (fig. 6), TSF thickness (fig. 7), and MUAMC (fig. 8) of children under 5 years of age were compared to Frisancho's percentiles. No Brazilian standards were available for comparison.

MUAC has been used as an indicator in identifying subjects who are malnourished. Results in this study indicated boys and girls generally had MUAC values near or above Frisancho's median values (50th percentile),

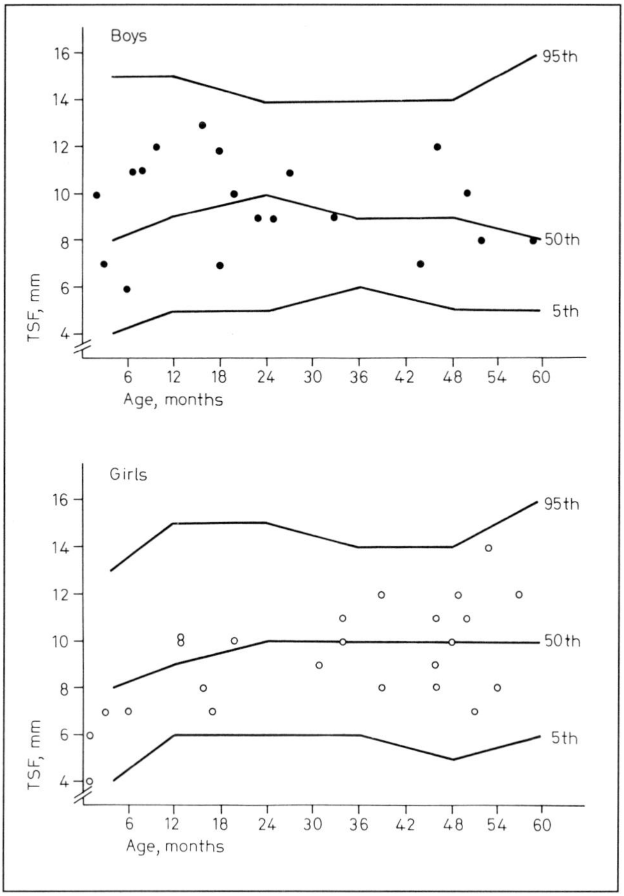

Fig. 7. Comparison of boys' and girls' TSF thickness with TSNS percentiles.

although some children had values approaching the 5th percentile. A few boys (10.5%) were probably malnourished as their MUAC values were below the 5th percentile.

Use of TSF thickness measurements, an indication of reserve energy stores as fat, demonstrated that children's TSF thickness values were generally satisfactory, with the majority of values near or above the median. Calculation of children's MUAMC values from TSF thickness and MUAC was conducted to determine adequacy of muscle development; an indication of the amount of protein reserves. When MUAMC values were com-

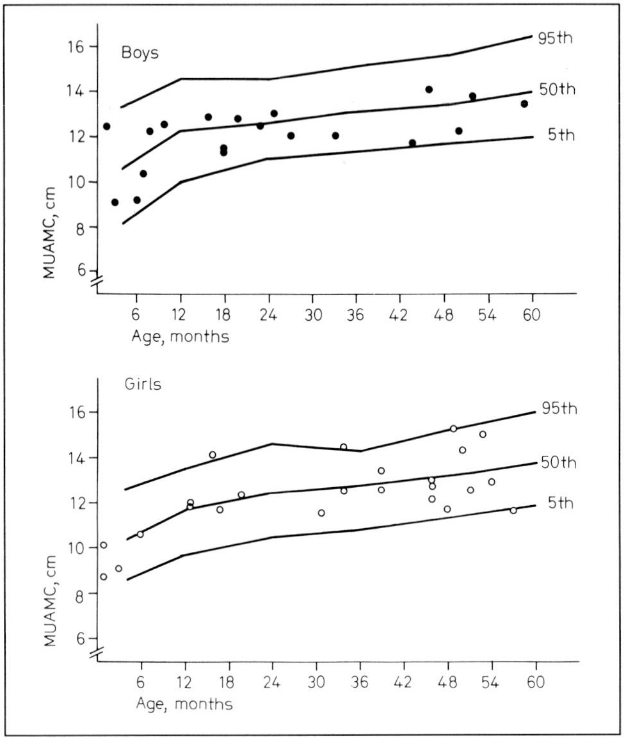

Fig. 8. Comparison of boys' and girls' MUAMC with TSNS percentiles.

pared to Frisancho's standards, most values for boys and girls were satisfactory, although a few subjects had values near or below the 5th percentile, implying that muscle development was poor.

Nutrition Knowledge and Attitudes, and Beliefs of Women

Nutrition Knowledge. Women (n = 56) were questioned to determine the degree of nutrition knowledge regarding reasons for eating a variety of foods, quantity of food to be consumed during pregnancy or lactation, and the types of foods beneficial and detrimental to newborns and young children. Results (table 14) indicated that the mean nutrition knowledge score was low (25.3% ± 9.9), with a range of scores from 4 to 60%. The majority of nutrition knowledge scores were below 50%, implying a low level of nutrition knowledge.

Table 14. Distribution of nutrition knowledge scores by women (figures express number and percent of respondents)

	Score, %	n	%
	<25	23	41.1
	25–49	27	48.2
	50–74	6	10.7
	75–100	0	0
Mean ± SD	25.3 ± 9.9		
Range	8–40		

Nutrition Attitudes/Beliefs. Women (n = 56) were questioned to determine their attitudes and beliefs regarding the origin of illness and consumption of special foods or food taboos during menstruation, pregnancy, lactation, and immediately post partum. Results indicated that a large percentage of respondents (37.3%) had no opinion regarding the origin of illness. A small number of respondents (16.8%), however, reported health and nutrition were implicated in illness, with contributing factors such as lack of food and consumption of contaminated water. Some women (13.6%) still believed in the hot/cold classification of disease; changes in weather, for example, were believed to cause illness.

Many respondents (69.6%) indicated that certain foods, such as cold food and beverages (i.e. cold in temperature), vegetables such as cabbage, onion, and red pepper, citrus fruits, acidic foods, and fish, should not be consumed during menstruation. Reasons most frequently cited for food taboos were that the foods caused headaches, upset stomach or resulted in cessation of menstrual flow. Fewer respondents (19.6%) reported food taboos during pregnancy; red pepper and alcoholic beverages were mentioned most frequently. Red pepper was believed to cause colic and red discoloration in infants; alcohol was believed to result in birth defects and discoloration in newborns. The majority of women (73.2%) also believed that certain foods, such as vegetables (onion, cabbage, red pepper, cucumber) and meat (fish, pork, other meat), should not be eaten immediately post partum. Vegetables were believed to cause illness and fever; meat was thought to cause colic, retention of water, and fissures of breast nipples. Furthermore, more than one third of respondents (37.5%) reported food taboos such as red pepper, meat, and fruit (oranges, pineapple) during lactation. Red pepper was thought to pass into breast milk and cause discoloration in the infant; meat was believed to cause allergies in the baby and reduce lactation; acidic fruits were thought to cause colic and make breast milk acidic.

Respondents were also asked whether any special foods were thought to be important during menstruation, pregnancy, post partum, and lactation. Only a small percentage of women (16.1%) believed certain foods such as rice, beans, and meat should be eaten especially during menstruation. More women thought that consumption of meat and fruit should be emphasized during pregnancy. Meat was believed to make the woman and baby strong; fruit was considered important for baby's nourishment and strength. More than one half of respondents (62.5%) also believed special foods such as soup and milk were important for the woman immediately post partum. Because women were considered weak immediately post partum, soup was thought to be nourishing; milk was reported to increase quantity of breast milk. Women (66.1%) also reported that special foods such as soup, milk, and meat were especially necessary during lactation, for nourishment and to increase the quantity of breast milk.

Overall, many food taboos during various physiological states were reported by women. Although no nutritionally detrimental food beliefs were reported during pregnancy, other taboos such as restriction of certain foods immediately post partum and during lactation could have potentially negative nutritional consequences for the mother and indirectly for the infant. Not all food beliefs, however, had negative nutritional consequences. Food taboos, such as alcohol consumption during pregnancy, for instance, as well as beliefs in the consumption of milk immediately post partum and intake of meat and milk during lactation have positive nutritional implications for the mother and baby.

In summary, evidence obtained from various sources such as the demographic/socioeconomic questionnaire, dietary intakes, anthropometry, nutrition knowledge scores, and nutrition attitudes and beliefs suggested that optimum health and nutrition probably did not exist for most Vila Diogo women and children. The existing poor economic situation, unhygienic physical environment, retarded growth in children, nutritionally detrimental infant feeding practices, and inadequate nutrient intakes would have negative nutritional consequences for this population, especially for nutritionally vulnerable groups such as children, pregnant and lactating women. Implementation of a nutrition education program for women (target group), emphasizing maximum use of available resources and importance of good nutrition practices on health and growth, appeared to be an appropriate nutrition intervention strategy for this population in these socioeconomic circumstances.

Nutrition Education Program Evaluation

Formative Evaluation

Written formative evaluations of nutrition education sessions were conducted after each session by instructors and primary investigator. Topics of evaluation included physical facilities, nutrition education material and presentation, instructors, and participants. The problems identified and appropriate action taken are described below.

Summative Evaluation

Summative evaluation of the nutrition education program included written evaluations by the primary investigator and instructors and statistical analysis of nutrition knowledge scores before and after completion of the program. Written evaluation discussed topics such as choice of location, weather, length of the program, participants, instructors, and educational material.

A 10-week nutrition education program, following an interview period of 2 months, was considered too long for this population. Participants and instructors were observed to be less enthusiastic and interested near the conclusion of the program.

Weather was an important consideration because sessions were generally held outdoors. Fall and early winter seemed most appropriate as weather was hot, with little precipitation. Nice weather, however, was a disadvantage for women field laborers who generally were unable to attend.

Other important considerations were size of location, location in the *favela,* personality of the hostess, as well as interpersonal relationships among women. Some of the locations selected were somewhat small for the number of participants present. One of the hostesses was shy and sometimes ill. Furthermore, after cancellation of one of the locations due to poor attendance, remaining sessions were held in one area of the *favela.*

Participation by women in the nutrition education program was fair (46.4%). Regular attendance was poor, with 53.9% of program participants attending less than one half of the weekly sessions. Average attendance was 8.5 ± 3.0 (range 2–15). A significant proportion of participants (26.9%), however, attended all sessions at least once a week. Furthermore,

Table 15. Comparison of women's nutrition knowledge scores pre- and post-nutrition education program

	Scores[a]		Difference[b]
	pre-program	post-program	
	10	15	+5
	2	6	+4
	10	20	+10
	7	6	−1
	3	4	+1
	9	8	−1
	8	19	+11
	9	12	+3
	9	11	+2
	6	12	+6
	4	15	+11
	7	3	−4
	5	13	+8
	4	3	−1
	4	11	+7
	7	6	−1
	5	11	+6
	5	2	−3
Mean	6.3 ± 2.5	9.8 ± 5.4	4.7 ± 3.5
Range	2–10	2–20	−4 to +11

[a] Based on maximum score of 25.

[b] Differences in pre- and post-program nutrition knowledge scores were statistically significant at $\alpha = 0.05$, using Wilcoxon signed ranks test.

some participants (42.3%) had attended at least one session more than once a week.

Women who participated in the nutrition education program, generally, were older (mean 43.0 years ± 15.6; range 19–77 years) than nonparticipants (mean 37.7 years ± 13.9; range 16–68 years). More than one third of participants were past the age of childbearing or lived alone. Children attended sessions regularly and were enthusiastic participants.

A few women who attended sessions were talkative and participated readily; others were timid, although some women gradually became more involved in later sessions. Participants had difficulty in remembering past sessions and required continual review and repetition of material.

In conclusion, barriers that appeared to affect participation and attendance in the nutrition program were weather (i.e. no rainfall), lack of interest or motivation, mental incompetency of a few women, illness, and negative interpersonal relationships among women. Motivating factors for women's participation may have been primarily for social interaction or to have a change from the home environment, with the desire to improve the family's situation or welfare as a less important factor.

A comparison of nutrition knowledge scores before and after the nutrition education program (table 15) showed that two thirds of post nutrition education program scores had improved. For scores showing no improvement, decrease in nutrition knowledge scores was minimal.

Statistical analysis of women's nutrition knowledge scores ($n = 18$) before and after the nutrition education program was conducted to determine whether the program had any significant effect on nutrition knowledge. Wilcoxon signed ranks test was used on subjects' nutrition knowledge scores, with results reported in table 15. Statistical analysis revealed that differences in scores were significant at $\alpha = 0.05$.

Discussion

Findings from this study are compared, when possible, with findings from other relevant studies. Demographic and socioeconomic characteristics of the study population such as housing characteristics, food and health related practices, as well as women's attitudes/beliefs regarding food, infant feeding practices, dietary intakes, and anthropometry of women and children are compared to previous Brazilian studies of urban agricultural migrants or low socioeconomic groups. In addition, dietary intakes and anthropometric results are compared to international recommendations or standards.

Demographic and Socioeconomic Characteristics of Vila Diogo Residents

Household Size. Household size in Vila Diogo may be considered large, with about 50% of households reporting more than four persons per household. Whether the trend of having large families in Vila Diogo will continue, considering the number of women currently practising family planning, is not known. With Brazil's economic problems on one hand, and the economic value of large families in low socioeconomic groups on the other hand, it seems that *Boias-Frias* will continue to have large families. Furthermore, when women were asked what family size they currently regarded as appropriate, about 50% of respondents stated that families should be the same size as they had, with more than 25% of women indicating a larger family size.

Literacy Rate and Level of Education. Literacy rate and education level among Vila Diogo residents were low, with 33.9% of male and 45.0% of female household heads having no formal education. For *Boias-Frias* receiving formal education, maximum schooling was 3 or 4 years. Furthermore, the number of male household heads reporting 3 or 4 years of schooling was 1.5 times greater than female household heads. Similar differences between male and female household heads' literacy rates were also observed. Reasons for adults not receiving more than 4 years of schooling may be that *fazenda* schools did not offer higher grades, lack of interest by *Boias-Frias,* or lack of school facilities.

Of more concern is that less than one half of Vila Diogo school age children were currently attending school. Reasons most frequently cited for children not attending school were that children were employed or children disliked school. Families probably still regard children as important contributors to family income. With a poor educational background, children in later life will probably have a similar occupation and socioeconomic status as their parents.

Research findings indicate a positive correlation between health and nutrition and the amount of formal education [Daly et al., 1979]. Reasons postulated for this positive correlation may be that increasing education results in better personal hygiene, improved child rearing, adoption of better diets, increased income to buy more food, to cite a few [Daly et al., 1979].

Residential History. Vila Diogo was a well-established *favela* with a relatively stable population. Mean years of residency in the present home was 6.3 years, which did not include time spent in the same *favela,* but in another house. Furthermore, 25% of respondents were born and raised in Vila Diogo.

Migration in this population consisted primarily of relatively short distances; from Nuporanga or surrounding *fazendas* and cities. Reasons for residential changes within the *favela* may have been to obtain a more favorable location or house. Motives most frequently cited for moving to Vila Diogo were to earn more money and to obtain better medical services. Families previously living on *fazendas,* for instance, probably had limited access to health and education services. Furthermore, the possibility of earning more money as a seasonal agricultural laborer than a regular wage on a *fazenda* may have been the motivating factor in changing place of residency. The reason for moving to the *favela* from Nuporanga was probably economic, as rent and perhaps taxes for village services were likely beyond their means.

Employment. Employment stability is a major concern for *Boias-Frias.* Their earning power as agricultural laborers is dependent on factors such as weather, good health, amount of work performed, and good crops. Although a minimum wage exists in Brazil, this does not apply to *Boias-Frias.*

Sick benefits are also not available. Health status for *Boias-Frias,* then, becomes very important in terms of potential income. Presence of helminthic infestation, inadequate diet in terms of energy and nutrients, infection, or poor health would decrease a laborer's physical capabilities, resulting in less work performed and less income. Several studies among physical laborers [Angeleli et al., 1983; Wolgemuth et al., 1982] have shown that dietary supplementation increased work performance.

Furthermore, many Vila Diogo households (62.5%) consisted of one wage earner. In these instances, if the wage earner is in poor health and has inadequate dietary intake which results in absenteeism from work or reduced work output, the consequences on the family could be nutritionally detrimental. An investigation of wages revealed that earnings for *Boias-Frias* were generally lower than current minimum wage.

Weather and crop yields are additional crucial factors affecting income. Rainfall not only prevents *Boias-Frias* from working in the fields, but excessive precipitation can be detrimental to crop yields. In 1983, excessive rainfall caused low cotton crop yields, resulting in less income for *Boias-Frias* who harvested the crops. Rain also prevents agricultural laborers from working in the fields, resulting in less income.

Housing Characteristics. A comparison of housing characteristics between rural Vila Diogo and the urban *favela* of Vila Recreio described by Swann [1979] indicates that perhaps housing conditions for Vila Diogo residents may have been somewhat better than their urban counterparts.

Although many Vila Diogo houses had earthen floors and insufficient number of windows for adequate lighting and ventilation, the size of houses, as determined by the number of rooms, was larger than reported for Vila Recreio. Furthermore, more Vila Diogo households had piped-in water than Vila Recreio, although the number of households with electricity was slightly less. Finally, all Vila Diogo respondents reported owning their own home, compared to 77% in Vila Recreio [Swann, 1979].

Sanitation in Vila Diogo was poor, the situation being similar to conditions reported by Swann [1979] and Waddell [1981] for Vila Recreio. Sewage disposal consisted of open gutters; garbage was usually disposed openly on yards or street, and toilet facilities were primarily yards or open gutters.

The unhygienic environment is an important factor affecting nutritional status, especially in children. Several Vila Diogo children, during the study, were admitted to hospital for removal of heavy worm loads such as *Ascaris lumbricoides.* Other parasitic infestations found among Vila Diogo residents, as reported by the local doctor, were *Giardia lamblia, Ancylostoma duodenal* or *braziliense, Tenia saginata* or *solium,* and *Strongyloides stercoralis.* Prevalence of parasitic infestation in Vila Diogo children is probably similar to a 60% infestation rate reported by Swann [1979] for Vila Recreio children. Improvements in sanitation would exert significant effects in improving nutritional status of Vila Diogo residents, especially in young children.

Women's Reproductive History. In this study, range of values for age at first menstruation varied from 10 to 17 years. Upper range of values for age at first menstruation may possibly have indicated the influence of poor nutrition. Malnutrition can affect biological maturation, manifesting itself in delayed onset of menarche [Anderson et al., 1981; Beaton and Patwardhan, 1976].

A large percentage of respondents reported abortions, stillbirths, and infant deaths. Poor nutrition may be implicated as an underlying cause in the high percentage of fetal wastage reported by Vila Diogo women. Pregnancy is a physiological state requiring increased nutrients for growth of maternal and fetal tissues [Iyengar, 1975].

Animal studies have shown that nutrient deficiencies can result in fetal wastage and growth retardation in animals [Iyengar, 1975]. In humans, Antonov [1947] found that physical hard work, mental stress, cold temperatures, and starvation in pregnant women during the siege of

Leningrad resulted in an unusually high number of premature births, stillbirths, and high infant morbidity and mortality rates. A study of pregnant Gambian women by Thomson et al. [1966] found that strenuous physical labor and inadequate dietary intake resulted in weight loss during pregnancy and statistically nonsignificant reductions in birth weights.

Another reason for the occurrence of stillbirths in the past could be due to fetal distress which might have been prevented by adequate medical care. Prior to the opening of Nuporanga hospital in 1965, infants were delivered in *favela* homes by Vila Diogo women.

Mean birth interval (2.3 years) was calculated for respondents with more than one child under 5 years of age. Current birth intervals are perhaps greater than in the past because many women use oral contraceptives. Religion does not appear to exert any influence in family planning decisions, even though most respondents indicated Roman Catholicism as their religion.

A review by Huffman [1984] of studies conducted in developing countries reported that birth intervals less than 1–2 years as being detrimental to the nutritional status of mother and child. This view is shared by Wishik and Stern [1972] who state that for women from low socioeconomic groups, a birth interval of one year still probably constitutes a nutritional risk for mother and child.

In summary, characteristics of this rural population, such as large household size, low literacy rates and educational levels, low income, lack of job security and an unhygienic physical environment, are indicators that individuals, especially children, are unlikely to exhibit optimum health and nutrition. Studies of other agricultural migrant workers with similar demographic and socioeconomic characteristics [Swann, 1979; Waddell, 1981] confirm these observations.

Food- and Health-Related Practices

Food-Related Practices. Meal patterns of Vila Diogo households were similar to those reported by Swann [1979] and Waddell [1981] for Vila Recreio, with breakfast usually consisting of coffee (with sugar) and perhaps bread; lunch and supper consisting of rice, beans, and sometimes a vegetable or salad. Many Vila Diogo women used gas as a cooking fuel, with an equal number of women using either wood or a combination of wood and gas. Although women reported walking long distances to gather wood at no cost, the economic advantages realized were important because the price of cooking gas doubled in June 1983.

Food costs for Vila Diogo families were probably comparatively less than reported by Swann [1979] for Vila Recreio. Food prices in Vila Recreio stores were an estimated 18% higher than in Ribeirao Preto city. Although food costs for Vila Diogo families may have been higher than Ribeirao Preto city, the difference was probably not 18%. Vila Diogo residents, therefore, may have economic advantages regarding food costs compared to their urban counterparts. Furthermore, many Vila Diogo households reported having some home-grown foods, unlike Vila Recreio households, who generally did not have gardens [Swann, 1979].

Changes in dietary habits were reported by about one half of women who had migrated to Vila Diogo. Milk was the item most frequently reported as being consumed at the previous location, but not in Vila Diogo because of price. For households who previously lived on *fazendas,* milk was probably obtained free or at very low costs. Women now, however, reported eating vegetables, meat (including organ meat such as liver), and bread in Vila Diogo; foods which had not been as readily available at their former location. For many women, residential changes resulted in the availability of a more varied diet, however, in exchange for deleting a nutritious food such as milk.

In summary, although food intakes are similar between rural *Boia-Fria* women in this study and urban *Boia-Fria* women described by Swann [1979], rural residents may have economic advantages compared to their urban counterparts regarding cooking fuel, food costs, and availability of fresh, home-grown vegetables.

Health-Related Practices. Alcohol consumption among *favela* residents in this study was a problem, particularly among men. This finding was also observed by Desai et al. [1980] in urban *favela* dwellers. Women, generally, reported a dislike of alcoholic beverages, although one or two women may have had a drinking problem.

Smoking prevalence was higher among male and female household heads in Vila Diogo than reported by Desai et al. [1980] for urban *favela* dwellers of Vila Recreio. In Vila Diogo, more than 1.5 times as many men smoked as women, implying perhaps that smoking by women may not be as acceptable in Brazilian culture. Some young children smoked, although prevalence was difficult to determine because parents were often unaware of children's smoking practices.

The amount of money or percent of income spent on alcohol and cigarettes is not known; furthermore, accurate information regarding alcohol and smoking expenditures is frequently difficult to obtain. Money used in purchasing alcohol or cigarettes, however, could be used to purchase a larger quantity or variety of food supplies.

Nutritional Assessment

Dietary Intakes of Women. Although *Boia-Fria* women indicated a preference for a variety of foods, the actual diets on a daily basis were simplistic, consisting primarily of rice, beans, and coffee with sugar. The majority of respondents would consume meat, cheese, macaroni, fruit (such as avocado, banana, tangerine), soft drinks, ice cream, and vegetables, such as sweet potato or manioc, on a weekly or less frequent basis.

In this study, the main reason postulated for differences observed between women's food preferences and frequency of food consumption is economic. Evidence supporting this postulation is that almost one third of women surveyed regarding what they would do or buy on winning the lottery indicated increasing the quantity of food purchased. The majority of women, however, indicated they would buy the same type of food currently purchased, but in larger quantity; about 25% of respondents reported they would buy more meat. That income is probably a major limiting factor in obtaining nutritionally adequate diets among Brazilian low income groups has been reported by others [Patrick and Simoes, 1971; Jansen et al., 1977; Ward and Amoni, 1980].

A diet consisting primarily of rice, beans, and coffee with sugar would not be expected to contain all the nutrients for good nutrition. This was verified by Swann [1979] who conducted dietary studies among *Boias-Frias* living in Vila Recreio, an urban favela of Ribeirao Preto city. Other studies [Basta, 1977; Jansen et al., 1977; Ward and Amoni, 1980; Thomas, 1982] reported, however, that nutrient intakes in rural areas were superior to urban centers.

Mean daily nutrient intakes of *Boia-Fria* women in this study were estimated using the 24-hour recall method. Since a previous study by Desai et al. [1980] reported that dietary intakes of *Boias-Frias* usually were different on Sundays, some interviews were conducted in this study to obtain dietary information for that particular day.

The 24-hour recall method has several limitations which have previously been discussed. Limitations such as memory and lack or representativeness of usual intake may be a lesser problem in *Boia-Fria* diets because of diet simplicity and similarity from day to day. Problems, however, such as accurately estimating serving size, overestimating portion sizes when intakes are low, or underestimating intake in expectation of receiving aid, could occur [Burk and Pao, 1980]. The 24-hour recall method, itself, tends to underestimate intakes [Burk and Pao, 1980].

In comparing estimated mean daily nutrient intakes with intakes of *Boia-Fria* women living in an urban *favela,* Vila Recreio [Swann, 1979], results indicated that energy and nutrient intakes (except ascorbic acid) of *Boia-Fria* women in this study were higher. Estimated mean daily intakes of protein, fat, thiamin, riboflavin, and niacin were about 1.5 times and vitamin A was 4 times greater in Vila Diogo women than in Vila Recreio women.

Estimated mean vitamin A intakes for subjects in this study, however, were probably not indicative of usual intake because a few subjects had consumed foods high in vitamin A. Furthermore, foods rich in vitamin A were not generally eaten on a daily basis. Foods high in a particular nutrient such as vitamin A are, therefore, not accurately portrayed by the 24-hour recall method because of daily nutrient variability [Beaton, 1975]. Standard deviations varied greatly for mean protein, calcium, vitamin A, riboflavin, and ascorbic acid intakes. Mean values for these nutrients are, therefore, more prone to error in estimating true population means.

Estimated mean daily intakes of women were compared to FAO recommended intakes. Almost two thirds and about one tenth of women surveyed did not meet two thirds and one third of FAO recommendations, respectively, for energy intake. Energy intakes in this study population were higher than reported by Swann [1979] for women living in Vila Recreio.

Regarding nutrient intake, fewer Vila Diogo women than their urban counterparts in Vila Recreio did not meet one third FAO recommendations for calcium, iron, riboflavin, and niacin, although the proportion of women not meeting one third of FAO recommended intakes for vitamin A and ascorbic acid were similar. Despite allowances for interindividual variation in collection of dietary data, it appears that intakes of energy and most nutrients are superior among women living in this rural *favela* than compared to women in the urban *favela* studied by Swann [1979].

The contribution of various food groups to nutrient intakes were relatively similar for Vila Diogo women and for urban *Boia-Fria* women described by Swann [1979]. Energy sources were provided primarily by legumes (beans) and cereals (rice). Regarding protein intake, however, Vila Diogo women had more protein intake than their urban counterparts from animal and legume sources. Calcium intakes were similar for both groups of women, primarily from legumes and cereals, and a small amount from dairy products. Iron sources were largely from legumes, ascorbic acid was primarily obtained from vegetables, α-tocopherol from legumes and cereals, and most thiamin, riboflavin, and niacin were obtained from animal sources, legumes, and cereals. Compared to Vila Recreio women, more vitamin A intake for Vila Diogo women originated from animal sources and less from vegetable sources. This may be due to the location of a chicken hatchery, abattoir, and meat shops in the vicinity of Vila Diogo.

Interpretation of Dietary Data. Interpretation of dietary data, whether for individuals or population groups, is difficult. Dietary data are usually compared to standards. Intakes below recommended levels, however, do not necessarily imply a deficiency [Health and Welfare Canada, 1983].

Standards have been derived from average requirements plus two standard deviations which will meet the needs of most healthy persons in a population [Health and Welfare Canada, 1983]. Recommended intakes exceed requirements of most individuals, with few individuals requiring nutrient levels recommended by dietary standards. Population groups, therefore, with mean nutrient intakes below recommended levels may only have a few individuals who are actually deficient in specific nutrients [Scrimshaw, 1962; Committee on Food Consumption Patterns, 1981]. Because dietary standards or allowances are derived from requirements of a healthy population, the presence of pathological conditions (which would increase nutrient requirements) such as infection, parasitic infestation, trauma, psychological stress, genetic abnormalities, and neoplastic disease are not taken into account [Scrimshaw, 1962].

Researchers have frequently compared dietary intakes to two thirds of recommended levels and used this value as a cut-off point for adequacy and inadequacy, although other cut-off points have been used [Burk and Pao, 1980]. Beaton [1975], however, proposes that assessment of nutrient intake be regarded as the probability of deficiency risk rather than inadequacy. Intakes below recommended levels would indicate a possible greater risk that an individual or population groups have not met their requirements [Health and Welfare Canada, 1983].

Estimated mean daily protein intake of Vila Diogo women met FAO recommendations, although the large standard deviation indicated significant error in the mean value as being the 'true' population mean. When individual protein intakes were compared with two thirds and one third of FAO recommendations, approximately 33 and 5% of women did not meet two thirds and one third of FAO levels, respectively.

Energy intake is one of the factors, however, that must be considered in determining the risk of protein deficiency. If energy intake is low, protein will be utilized for energy. In this study, mean daily energy intake was less than recommended, with almost 67% and more than 10% of women, respectively, not meeting two thirds and one third of FAO energy recommendations. A few women could, therefore, be at significant risk for protein deficiency and malnutrition if low intakes (less than one third of FAO levels) were continued. Other factors, furthermore, that can increase protein requirements include amino acid composition, protein digestibility, illness, trauma, infection, and physiological conditions such as lactation and pregnancy [Harper, 1982].

Protein sources of *Boia-Fria* diets are predominantly legumes and cereals. It has been suggested that in low-income populations where protein sources are mainly of plant origin (i.e. poorer protein quality) and where a higher probability of infection and malabsorption exists, that protein intake should be 13–14% of total energy intake to ensure adequate coverage of most people [Scrimshaw and Lockwood, 1980]. In this study, estimated mean protein intake accounted for 11% of total energy intake. Protein quality of the *Boia-Fria* rice and beans diet will be satisfactory, if consumed on a one-to-one ratio because the limiting amino acid of lysine in rice and methionine in beans are complemented. Protein status of Vila Diogo women may be marginal, with some women being at high risk for protein deficiency if pregnant, lactating, or ill.

Calcium intakes of Vila Diogo women were low, with almost 50% of women reporting intakes less than one third FAO recommendations. Furthermore, the standard deviation for estimated mean daily calcium intake was high, indicating a significant error in estimating the 'true' population mean. Daily calcium absorption may range from 10 to 60% although the body regulates calcium levels through urinary and fecal excretion, hormones, intestinal absorption, renal reabsorption, and bone resorption [Avioli, 1980; Robinson, 1980].

Low calcium intakes have been reported as well in other Brazilian low-income groups [Jansen et al., 1977; Swann, 1979]. Vila Diogo women appear to be at some risk for calcium deficiency, especially during periods of increased requirements such as pregnancy and lactation.

Iron intakes by Vila Diogo women appear very low, with about 90 and 50% of women not meeting two thirds and one third of FAO recommended levels, respectively. Occurrence of iron deficiency anemia would be expected in a small percentage of women, with a large percentage of women at high risk for developing anemia. Biochemical studies by Swann [1979] of *Boia-Fria* women in Vila Recreio found about 25% had low hemoglobin values.

Iron sources for Vila Diogo women were similar to Vila Recreio women, being obtained primarily from nonheme sources such as beans and rice. Iron bioavailability from nonheme sources is low (1–5%), although dietary ascorbic acid and heme sources would increase iron absorption. Cooking utensils used by Vila Diogo women did not add to iron intake, although drinking water may have provided additional small amounts of ingested iron. Mean estimated amounts of iron absorbed may, therefore, be very low compared to FAO recommendations.

Furthermore, increased iron loss such as sweating, however, could be important factors influencing iron status for women working as field laborers. Menstrual losses could result in substantial iron loss, although many Vila Diogo women of child-bearing age used oral contraceptives. Finally, parasitic infestation could account for iron loss, although prevalence of parasites such as hookworm in adult *Boias-Frias* was not known. Although iron absorption in iron-deficient individuals increases (ranging from 10 to 20%) [Beutler, 1980], subjects in this study are probably still at a high risk for developing iron deficiency anemia because increased iron absorption by the body will be insufficient to cover low dietary iron intake and iron losses.

Estimated mean daily vitamin A intakes of Vila Diogo women were very low, with about 90 and 73% of women not meeting two thirds and one third of FAO recommended vitamin A intakes, respectively. Furthermore, standard deviation was high, indicating the estimated mean value of vitamin A intake was an inaccurate estimation of the true population mean. This result was explained by a few subjects reporting consumption of foods high in vitamin A.

Considering that intakes of vitamin-A-rich foods among Vila Diogo women occurs infrequently, vitamin A liver reserves would probably be low or exhausted. Biochemical studies by Swann [1979] of Vila Recreio adults (male and female) found that 25% of subjects examined had low plasma vitamin A levels, indicating that vitamin A liver reserves were probably exhausted. Other studies of low socioeconomic groups, especially in northeastern Brazil, have also found vitamin A intakes to be low [ICNND, 1965; Patrick and Simoes, 1971; Ward and Amoni, 1980].

Estimated mean daily intake of ascorbic acid in Vila Diogo women was less than one half of FAO recommendations, with more than 65% of women not meeting one third of FAO recommended intakes. Similar findings were reported by Swann [1979] for Vila Recreio women, although mean ascorbic acid intake was slightly higher compared to Vila Diogo women. Considering that usually dietary intakes of vegetables and fruits are low, Vila Diogo women are probably at relatively high risk for ascorbic acid deficiency. This risk is increased, furthermore, in women who smoke. Evidence has shown that for persons smoking less than 20 cigarettes per day, plasma ascorbic acid levels may be 25% lower than for nonsmokers [Health and Welfare Canada, 1983]. Ascorbic acid requirements for smokers would, therefore, be even greater.

Mean estimated daily α-tocopherol intake, of all nutrients, was closest in meeting FAO recommendations, with only 27 and 5.4% of women not meeting two thirds and one third of FAO recommendations, respectively. Intakes of α-tocopherol for Vila Diogo women were much higher than for Vila Recreio women, with the majority of intake derived from rich sources such as legumes and cereals, and a smaller portion originating from oils.

Plasma α-tocopherol levels of almost all Vila Recreio women were at acceptable levels. Plasma α-tocopherol levels of Vila Diogo women would be expected to be adequate, with risk of α-tocopherol deficiency, therefore, being negligible for most women.

Intakes of thiamin, riboflavin, and niacin were low, although thiamin and niacin intakes of Vila Diogo women were generally superior to reported intakes in Vila Recreio [Swann, 1979]. An explanation for low thiamin intake is that typical *Boia-Fria* diets are high in polished rice and low in meat. Riboflavin intake is very low because riboflavin-rich foods such as dairy and animal products are usually lacking in *Boia-Fria* daily intakes. Risk of riboflavin deficiency is, therefore, probably high. Niacin-rich sources are varied, including dairy products, animal protein, grains, and vegetables. A significant contributor of niacin for Vila Diogo women was coffee, which accounted for 13.1% of total niacin intake.

To summarize, *Boia-Fria* diets were simplistic, and nutritionally inadequate. Low income appeared to be a major limiting factor in obtaining nutritionally adequate diets. The risk of nutrient deficiency in Vila Diogo women appeared to be greater in vitamin A, iron, calcium, ascorbic acid, and riboflavin.

Recommended Dietary Improvements. Any recommendations for dietary improvements should consider the cultural background and income of subjects, and physical availability of food. Furthermore, suggested dietary improvements should build on the existing positive elements of the diet.

Staple foods of Brazilian diets are beans, rice, and coffee (consumed with sugar). Although many varieties of beans exist in Brazil, about 20 varieties are mainly used for consumption, with certain varieties of beans being more popular in different geographical areas [Francois and Sizaret, 1981].

In recent years, Brazilian production of beans has not met consumption demand. The most common problem in increasing domestic production of beans is that any available arable land is used for export crops such as soybeans, coffee, and sugar [Francois and Sizaret, 1981]. Furthermore, attempts to introduce soybeans into *Boia-Fria* diets have been relatively unsuccessful due to soybean's taste and cooking qualities [Wright et al., 1982].

The staple diet of rice and beans has been described as ideal, especially for low-income groups who cannot afford daily intakes of animal protein [Francois and Sizaret, 1981]. Shortages of energy and protein intake by Vila Diogo women could probably be met, income permitting, by increasing quantity of rice and bean consumption. If availability of beans becomes more of a problem in the future, more people might switch to less nutritious wheat products such as macaroni [Francois and Sizaret, 1981].

Another serious concern is the lack of vegetables and fruits in diets of Vila Diogo women. Physical availability of a variety of fresh fruit and vegetables in Nuporanga stores is relatively low and probably too expensive for Vila Diogo residents. Women may rely more on local truck vendors for vegetables of better quality and price. Many Vila Diogo women have home gardens to some extent, and these attempts at domestic food production should be encouraged, as well as emphasizing consumption of locally grown fruit.

Consumption of dairy products among Vila Diogo women is low. Of the dairy products available, fresh milk would be the most economical. Lactose intolerance in *Boias-Frias* has not been reported to be a problem [Desai et al., 1980], and increasing milk consumption should, therefore, be encouraged. Milk consumption would be especially beneficial in increasing energy, protein, vitamin A, and riboflavin intakes.

Availability of organ meat in Nuporanga was probably greater than in the small Vila Recreio stores. Contrary to previous reports [Desai et al., 1980], organ meat such as liver is not totally rejected in *Boia-Fria* diets because some intake was reported in Vila Diogo. Because the price of organ meat is presumably less than other meat and because of its nutritional value, intakes of organ meat should be emphasized. Although consumption of poultry is infrequent, the Brazilian practice of incorporating chicken blood into the cooking of poultry should be encouraged.

Coffee with sugar is regarded by Brazilians as an important cultural beverage. This beverage cannot be totally disregarded as a nonnutritious food because coffee provided a significant proportion of niacin intake. Sugar used by *Boias-Frias* in this study was not very refined and could, therefore, contain some trace minerals.

Enrichment and fortification of Brazilian foods such as bread and macaroni have often been suggested. This suggestion, however, does not appear realistic for the Vila Diogo population because consumption of these foods is infrequent due to cost and perhaps some degree of cultural unacceptability.

In conclusion, Vila Diogo women should be encouraged to consume more fresh fruit and vegetables, dairy products, and organ meats. Families, for instance, could be encouraged to grow more produce. Government programs for food enrichment or fortification, such as enriched wheat products (e.g. bread, macaroni), would be of little value to this population who, financially, are unable to purchase these items on a regular basis.

Dietary Intakes of Children (2–5 years). When dietary intakes of Vila Diogo children were compared to women's intakes, a larger percentage of children met FAO energy and nutrient recommendations, especially for energy, protein, thiamin, and riboflavin. Estimated mean intakes for iron were low, with nonheme sources such as beans being the primary source. Estimated mean ascorbic acid intake was also low due to lack of fruit and vegetable consumption. A large standard deviation for estimated mean vitamin A intake indicated that although mean intake was higher than FAO recommendations, a few subjects had consumed vitamin-A-rich foods. Mean calcium intake appeared satisfactory, due primarily to milk consumption, although a relatively large standard deviation implied that some children had consumed little or no milk during the time period surveyed. Estimated mean protein intakes generally met FAO recommendations, with intakes being about equally derived from meat, rice and milk. The source of energy intake was primarily from rice. Milk consumption accounted for the satisfactory intakes of thiamin and riboflavin, and a significant proportion of all vitamin A intake.

Considering that children's nutrient requirements are high due to rapid growth, inadequate nutrient intakes plus other factors, such as infections, illness, or parasitic infestation, could adversely affect growth and health. Comparison of estimated mean energy and nutrient intakes with FAO recommendations indicate that one third of children had mean energy and riboflavin intakes and one half of children had calcium, iron and α-tocopherol intakes less than two thirds of FAO recommendations, with more than three quarters of children not meeting two thirds of FAO levels for vitamin A, niacin, and ascorbic acid. One quarter and one half of children had mean vitamin A and ascorbic acid intakes, respectively, less than one third of FAO recommendations.

A number of children may have been at some risk regarding low energy intakes, although a proportion of protein intake may have been used for energy purposes. Children, generally, would appear to be at high risk for developing iron deficiency anemia, for having low liver vitamin A reserves, if any, and for being deficient in ascorbic acid.

Improvements in dietary intake are similar to those suggested for Vila Diogo women. Suggested changes include increasing energy intake, milk consumption, fruit, dark green and yellow vegetables, and heme iron sources (organ meat, other meat). Dietary improvements are necessary if catch-up growth is to occur in children who are stunted in growth.

Infant Feeding Practices in Vila Diogo. All children under the age of 5 years who participated in this study had been breast-fed at birth. A general trend in developing countries, however, is a decline in breast-feeding, especially in urban centers [WHO, 1981a].

A study conducted in Pelotas, a southern Brazilian city, found that 24.0% of infants from low socioeconomic families were not breast-fed at birth [Sousa et al., 1975]. Furthermore, studies in southern Brazil indicated that the majority of infants had been weaned by the second month [Sousa et al., 1975; Schmidt et al., 1980]. In the present study, 63.1% of infants had already been weaned by the third month.

A comparison of weaning practices in Vila Diogo with Vila Recreio revealed 73.6% of Vila Diogo infants had been weaned after 6 months, compared to 30% for Vila Recreio infants [Desai et al., 1980]. At the end of 18 months, all infants in this study had been weaned. Differences noted in weaning practices between subjects in this study and those reported by Desai et al. [1980] are contrary to general trends reported in the literature of declining weaning age in rural and especially urban low socioeconomic groups. Differences in weaning age between Vila Diogo and Vila Recreio infants could be due to the presence of more working mothers in Vila

Diogo than Vila Recreio. It is assumed that working women (e.g. field laborers) would terminate breast feeding at an earlier age compared to women who are not employed. Furthermore, Nuporanga State Health Post offered free milk powder to Vila Diogo infants who were not growing well. This may have provided an incentive for women to terminate breast-feeding at an earlier age. Distribution of free milk powder to Vila Recreio infants has not been reported.

The breast milk supplement or substitute used by majority of women was powdered milk. Since illiteracy among women was high, directions for preparation of milk were probably not known nor followed. Furthermore, the cost factor may have resulted in women preparing milk of a weaker strength. Other problems mentioned in the literature regarding infant formula preparation in developing countries are the lack of facilities for cleaning bottles, improper technique, and unhygienic environment, resulting in highly contaminated infant formulas [WHO, 1981a].

Practices of introducing nonmilk foods in Vila Diogo appear more favorable than those reported by Desai et al. [1980] for Vila Recreio. Sugar water, coffee (with sugar), and soft drinks were not introduced to infants' diets during the first month of life, although 25% of infants were given herb tea (with sugar). In contrast, 80% of Vila Recreio women reported feeding infants sugar water and herb tea (with sugar) during the first week of life; 60% of Vila Recreio women were feeding infants gruel (manioc flour or cornstarch and water), coffee (with sugar), and soft drinks within 2 weeks of birth. In Vila Diogo, only a small percentage of women used gruel as a weaning food. General recommendations for infant feeding state that foods other than milk are not necessary until the third or fourth month of the infant's life [WHO, 1981a].

The age at which solid foods were introduced to Vila Diogo infants was similar to practices reported by Desai et al. [1980] for Vila Recreio. No solid foods, such as bread, vegetables, cereals, or meat, were given to infants less than one month of age; by one year of age, most infants were eating the regular family diet.

Infant feeding practices changed significantly during illness and were nutritionally detrimental. For infants with fever, many were only given liquids. The majority of mothers did not give infants anything to eat or drink, gave only liquids, or purges when infants had diarrhea.

Earlier thoughts on treatment of diarrhea involved fasting, thereby allowing the bowel to rest. Subsequent research, however, found that feeding did not increase duration of diarrhea, and nutrient absorption was still possible [Synderman, 1980]. These observations resulted in the recommendation of feeding during diarrhea. The use of starvation in treating infantile diarrhea among low socioeconomic groups in developing countries can be particularly detrimental for the infant's nutritional status, which may already have been less than optimum before diarrhea occurred.

Women's Attitudes and Beliefs Regarding Illness and Food. An investigation of food taboos and other beliefs regarding food and origin of illness found a significant number (30%) of women did not know what could cause illness, although more than 16% of respondents cited health-related reasons, such as insufficient food, drinking contaminated water, and an unhygienic environment. Belief in the 'hot-cold' theory of illness was still prevalent, with more than 20% of women reporting that changes in weather, consumption of cold (temperature) foods and drinks, or exposing one's hot body to the wind, could cause illness.

Many women reported that special foods, such as meat and fruit, as well as milk and vitamin supplements, were important during pregnancy for fetal nourishment. Women recognized and reported a relationship between maternal dietary intake and fetal nourishment. These observations are contrary to those reported by Desai et al. [1980] for Vila Recreio women, who indicated that no special foods were necessary during pregnancy and lactation.

Many food taboos reported by Vila Diogo women were related to the 'hot-cold' food classification still prevalent in Latin America. Illnesses or physiological conditions are classified as hot or cold, with treatment consisting of foods or medicaments opposite in classification [Sanjur, 1982]. Menstruation, pregnancy, lactation, and post partum are considered hot conditions, and hot foods such as cabbage, onions, beans, pork, cereals, alcohol, and peppers would be avoided [Harwood, 1971; Molony, 1975; Desai et al., 1980]. Examples of cold foods are oranges, herb tea, lettuce, milk, and tomato [Harwood, 1971; Molony, 1975; Desai et al., 1980].

The majority of women (75%) reported food taboos such as cold temperature foods and drinks, ice, meat (especially fish), red pepper, onions, cabbage, and acidic foods (citrus fruit) during menstruation. Whether women still rigidly adhere to these taboos is not known.

Fewer women reported food taboos during pregnancy. Reasons cited for taboos such as alcohol and red pepper were that pepper would cause colic or red color in the newborn; alcohol would cause birth defects or red color. A few women recognized the potential danger of maternal alcohol consumption on the fetus. Whether this knowledge was a result of attending prenatal classes was not investigated. These findings are contrary to those reported by Desai et al. [1980] for some Vila Recreio women who believed that hot foods such as rice, beans, onions were undesirable during pregnancy.

More than one third of Vila Diogo women reported taboos during lactation, such as red pepper, fish, other meat, and acidic fruits. Very few Vila Recreio women, however, reported food taboos during lactation [Desai et al., 1980].

Almost 75% of Vila Diogo women reported that a wide variety of foods should be avoided immediately post partum. Reasons for taboos were sometimes not known; however, some women stated food taboos were necessary because the mother was physically weak. These taboos, if observed, could be nutritionally detrimental to the mothers. With most deliveries now occurring in hospital, however, these taboos are probably no longer practised.

From findings reported by Desai et al. [1980], it seems that as *Boias-Frias* move to urban centers, fewer women may remember and/or practise various food taboos. Some modification of food taboos in Vila Diogo have probably already occurred as a result of most newborns being delivered in hospital rather than *favela* homes. With continued health education programs, such as prenatal classes, more potentially detrimental food taboos may be eventually rejected.

Anthropometric Status of Women. Mean height, weight, TSF, MUAC, and MUAMC of Vila Diogo women were similar to Vila Recreio women, as reported by Swann [1979]. Weight for height of Vila Diogo women were compared with NCHS percentiles. This index has been recommended as useful in indicating present nutritional level.

A large percentage of women (62.4%) had weight-for-height values below the NCHS median (50th percentile), with 25% below the 5th percentile. This would indicate that women are probably undernourished.

More than one third of Vila Diogo women (37.6%) had weight-for-height values at the 50th percentile or greater, implying normal or above-normal weights. A small percentage of women (6.3%) had weight-for-height values above the 90th percentile, indicating the presence of obesity. Overweight and obesity may occur as a result of excessive energy intake, insufficient exercise, metabolic disorders, or weight gain after successive pregnancies. In Vila Diogo, women who were obese usually were not agricultural laborers, but led a sedentary life-style. Garn and Clark, as reported by Richardson [1980], note a trend for low socioeconomic women to become more obese than women of higher socioeconomic groups.

TSF measurements of Vila Diogo women revealed that 10% had TSF values below the 5th percentile. Low TSF values indicate that little energy reserves, as fat, exist. A small percentage of women would probably have little subcutaneous fat for energy reserves.

Calculation of MUAMC, using TSF and MUAC values, can indicate the state of muscle development. Poor muscle development or muscle wasting indicates malnutrition, whereas a large muscle mass implies increased use of certain muscle groups [Jelliffe, 1966].

Muscle development was satisfactory for most Vila Diogo women, with 12.5 % of women having MUAMC values greater than the 95th percentile. No values were below the 5th percentile. The relatively large number of women with significant muscle development (greater than 95th percentile) is probably for women who were agricultural laborers.

Anthropometric Status in Children. Height, weight, and HC of Vila Diogo children under 5 years were compared to NCHS percentiles [derived from Health and Nutrition Examination Survey, HANES, 1971–1975] and Marcondes' 50th percentile (derived from a Sao Paulo survey, 1971). HANES data were obtained from a sample representative of the USA population by age, sex, race, income, and region; Marcondes' sample was derived primarily from low socioeconomic groups [Murphy and Michael, 1981; Marcondes et al., 1971]. Comparison of Vila Diogo children's anthropometric measurements with Brazilian standards would, therefore, present a more favorable image regarding growth because children from low socioeconomic groups would probably exhibit varying degrees of poor nutrition. Although use of local anthropometric reference standards are desirable, standards ideally should be developed using healthy, well-fed subjects from upper socioeconomic groups [Jelliffe, 1966].

When weight-for-age values of Vila Diogo boys and girls were compared to NCHS percentiles, 25% of boys and 10% of girls had weight-for-age values less than the 5th percentile. These results imply that numerous boys and a few girls could be undernourished. Weight-for-age index, however, overestimates the number of malnourished because the index does not account for children small for size [Richardson, 1980].

Weight-for-height index, on the other hand, considers weight in relation to frame size. When the weight-for-height index was used, 15.4% of boys and no girls had weight-for-height values below the 5th percentile; only a small percentage of boys, therefore, could probably be considered as undernourished.

Height-for-age index is an indicator of past nutrition. A large percentage of boys (46.2%) and girls (31.6%) had height-for-age values below the 5th percentile. A significant percentage of boys and girls could, therefore, be considered stunted. Stunting has been described as a physiological adaptation to low nutrient intake in an effort to conserve available energy [Richardson, 1980]. Whether these children will remain stunted in later life will depend on whether catch-up growth occurs, and to what degree. Reasons for stunting may include inadequate dietary intake, infection, parasitic infestation, or illness. The degree to which catch-up growth is completed will depend on the timing, degree, and duration of malnutrition [Fomon, 1974]. These results are similar to those found by Dorea et al. [1982] for preschool and school children in northeastern Brazil, where weight-for-height values were adequate, but where stunting (height for age) had occurred. From other anthropometric studies conducted in Brazilian children under 5 years of age, it appears that Vila Diogo children are better nourished than children in certain cities in northeastern and northern Brazil [Filho et al., 1981]. Stunting, observed in Vila Diogo children under 5 years of age, was also reported by Desai et al. [1981] for Vila Recreio children. Comparison of weight-for-age values between Vila Diogo and Vila Recreio children, however, seemed to indicate higher values, generally, for Vila Diogo children than for Vila Recreio children.

TSF thickness, MUAC, and calculated MUAMC values in Vila Diogo children were generally normal, indicating fairly adequate fat reserves and no muscle wasting. Although MUAC and MUAMC values for Vila Diogo and Vila Recreio children appeared similar, Vila Diogo children, generally, appeared to have higher TSF thickness measurements than in Vila Recreio children [Desai et al., 1981].

For Vila Diogo children less than 3 years of age, 62 and 15% of boys and 55 and 27% of girls had HC less than the 50th and 5th percentiles, respectively. Head growth occurs most rapidly during the first few years of life. Any nutritional deprivation would, therefore, be reflected in size of HC.

HC values of Vila Diogo children indicate that some nutritional deprivation has or is occurring. These observations are confirmed by comparing

50th percentiles of NCHS and Marcondes' references, where NCHS references are derived from healthy, relatively high socioeconomic groups compared to lower Marcondes' values derived from low socioeconomic groups that are probably nutritionally deprived.

Nutrition Education Program

Few reports of nutrition education programs among Brazilian low socioeconomic groups have been published. Wright [1982] used two education approaches (lecture and discussion/decision) to introduce soybeans into agricultural migrants' diets. Drummond [1975], using Freire's philosophy of education, conducted a nutrition education program in northeastern Brazil among low socioeconomic groups. Community meetings were held to discuss various health and nutrition problems existing in the communities.

In this study, nutrition education was considered the most appropriate nutrition intervention strategy in view of the limited research resources of time and finances and the demographic/socioeconomic characteristics of the study population. The low socioeconomic status of Vila Diogo residents, compounded by high national inflation, job insecurity, and lack of government programs to aid low socioeconomic groups, provided justification for implementing a nutrition education program that would focus attention, for example, on how people could maximize use of scarce resources. It has been reported that improving nutrition knowledge, using nutrition education, can be a means whereby the poor can learn how to achieve maximum benefits from limited resources [Al-Isi et al., 1975].

The 10 weeks allotted for the nutrition education program were recognized as too brief to expect changes in nutrition attitudes/beliefs and nutrition practices in Vila Diogo women (target group), but changes in nutrition knowledge were anticipated. Nutrition attitudes, beliefs, and practices are an integral part of culture and are subject to change even as culture, itself, changes. This change process, however, may be relatively slow.

Nutrition education's goal has often been erroneously regarded as only to change nutrition behavior or practices [Kolasa, 1981]. Nutrition education, however, may be used to emphasize or reinforce positive nutrition behavior currently practised by the target group. In Vila Diogo, evidence that all young children commenced breast feeding at birth, that many women had home gardens, and women's beliefs that alcohol consumption during pregnancy could be detrimental to the fetus were positive nutrition practices and beliefs that should be emphasized and reinforced. Other evidence, such as inadequate nutrient intake, nutritionally detrimental infant feeding practices, stunted growth in children, potentially nutritionally detrimental attitudes/beliefs and low nutrition knowledge scores, indicated that nutrition education topics, such as breast feeding, infant feeding practices during illness, importance of eating a variety of foods, and maximizing use of available resources, should be presented.

The philosophical approach to nutrition education in this study was the 'banking' method as described by Freire [1981]. A more desirable approach proposed by Freire [1981], where program participants would analyze their situation, identify problems, and suggest solutions, was not attempted in this study because time was limited, instructors were unfamiliar with this method, and the primary investigator had a limited command of the local language. This method, involving participants in the development and implementation of a nutrition education program, has been described as the most successful means of changing nutrition behavior [Gussow and Contento, 1984]. If this problem-solving approach were to be attempted with this population, discussions should involve male household heads as well as women. In Brazilian society, the male role is regarded as dominant. Program success might be assured if men were involved in problem identification and decision-making.

Overall participation by women in the nutrition education program was fair (46.4%). The mean age of women who participated was slightly higher than for nonparticipants (43.0 vs 37.7 years). Reasons postulated for nonparticipation were: 2 or 3 women were mentally incompetent, one woman was physically disabled, one woman refused to pass through the *favela,* and a number of women were field laborers who worked every day except Saturday (and may have been too busy or tired to attend). For the remaining women who did not participate, reasons were unknown.

Although many participants were older women, nutrition education may be valuable if older women are a source of information to their daughters. Some evidence that this might be true was revealed in reasons given for food taboos. In a few instances, the reason cited for a food taboo was that the elders had stated taboos were necessary or important.

Although women rather than children were the target group of nutrition education, children attended nutrition education sessions and were enthusiastic participants. Future nutrition education programs for low socioeconomic groups should, perhaps, consider including children as a target group. Involving children in appropriate nutrition education programs could affect children by increasing nutrition knowledge and possibly cause changes in nutritionally detrimental attitudes/beliefs and behaviors as children grow older and eventually have their own families.

Evaluation of the nutrition education program in Vila Diogo consisted of two components; formative and summative evaluation. Frequently, insufficient attention has been focused on formative evaluation. Advantages of evaluating programs during the implementation and operational phases are that any problems or shortcomings can be quickly identified and corrected during the program, preventing errors from recurring. In this study, formative evaluation was of value in identifying problems of attendance, length of sessions, manner of presentation, and participants' response.

Summative evaluation consisted of a written evaluation and statistical analysis of nutrition knowledge scores. Statistical analysis of nutrition knowledge scores before and after the nutrition education program, using Wilcoxon signed ranks test, indicated that improvement in scores was statistically significant at $\alpha = 0.05$.

Does statistical significance, however, necessarily imply any practical significance? Hennigan et al. [1979] state that even though changes may be statistically significant, changes may be too small to make any practical difference in people's lives. In this study, statistical significance in improved nutrition knowledge scores was unlikely to have any real effect on women's lives. Furthermore, bias created as a result of a large percentage of nonparticipants would prevent speculation that an increase in nutrition knowledge scores could be predicted for other similar populations. If one disregards the issue whether nutrition education had any practical significance for Vila Diogo women, and in spite of bias resulting from a large proportion of nonparticipants, nutrition education did result in improving nutrition knowledge for women who attended the program.

Summary and Recommendations

Summary

A nutritional needs assessment was conducted among rural agricultural migrant women (target group) and children (less than 5 years). The study was conducted in Vila Diogo, a slum located on the periphery of Nuporanga, a village in Sao Paulo state, Brazil.

A nutrition education program was designed on the basis of evidence obtained from demographic/socioeconomic information of the study population and a nutritional needs assessment of women (target group) and children less than 5 years of age. The nutritional needs assessment consisted of anthropometry, dietary assessment, and nutrition knowledge, attitudes, and beliefs questionnaires. Formative and summative evaluation of the nutrition education program, using appropriately selected criteria and comparisons of nutrition knowledge scores before and after the program, were used to determine program effectiveness.

Major findings of the study were: Diets of Vila Diogo residents were generally simplistic, consisting primarily of rice, beans, and coffee with sugar. Vila Diogo women appeared to be at a relatively high risk for vitamin A, iron, calcium, ascorbic, and riboflavin deficiencies, based on comparisons of 24-hour dietary intake data with FAO recommendations. Children (2–5 years) appeared at high risk for vitamin A, iron, and ascorbic acid deficiencies, based on comparisons of 24-hour dietary intake data with FAO recommendations. All children less than 5 years of age had been breast-fed at birth, but more than one half of children had been weaned by the third month.

Infant feeding practices during fever and diarrhea were nutritionally detrimental. Women generally recognized a relationship between dietary intake during pregnancy and fetal nourishment. Using weight-for-height index, a significant number of women were probably undernourished; a small percentage of women, however, were overweight or obese. Although children less than 5 years of age did not generally appear malnourished, a relatively large number were stunted in growth. Although Vila Diogo women reported many food taboos during various physiological states (menstruation, pregnancy, immediately post partum, lactation), relatively few food taboos had potentially negative nutritional consequences. For women who participated in the nutrition education program, nutrition knowledge scores after the program showed improvement which was statistically significant at $\alpha = 0.05$, using Wilcoxon signed rank test.

Recommendations

On the basis of results obtained from this study, the following recommendations for further investigation or action are presented: Comparing dietary intakes between rural and urban *Boias-Frias* during a similar time frame. Comparing the effectiveness of a nutrition education program between rural and urban *Boia-Fria* women. Designing and implementing a nutrition education program for *Boia-Fria* children. Comparing weaning age between rural and urban *Boia-Fria* children. Revising nutritional material used in this study to make it more appropriate for *Boias-Frias*. Investigating whether food attitudes/beliefs change, and to what extent, when *Boia-Fria* women move from a rural to an urban setting. Investigating decision-making within the home: how money is spent, who controls finances, who is involved in the decision-making process.

Investigating how food is distributed within the home. Comparing sources of health and nutrition information for *Boias-Frias* women living in rural and urban *favelas*. Investigating how additional income would actually be used compared to reported use. Investigating whether *Boia-Fria* men tend to marry *Boia-Fria* women and remain in the *favela;* whether *Boia-Fria* women tend to marry men other than *Boias-Frias* (to increase socioeconomic status), and the nutritional implications for adults and children. To encourage use of mass media (e.g. posters, television) by State Health Posts for promoting positive nutrition practices such as breast-feeding, cultivation of home gardens to cite a few. Using the methodology of Freire, to conduct a nutrition education program among *Boias-Frias* living in Sao Paulo state. Investigating reasons for women engaging in positive nutrition practices such as breast-feeding, family planning, and cultivating home gardens, and using this information in planning future nutrition intervention programs.

Acknowledgements

The authors would like to acknowledge the following individuals and institutions for their generous support and valuable contributions towards this research project: Fundaçao de Amparo a Pesquisa do Estado de Sao Paulo (FAPESP); International Scientific Exchange Program of the Natural Sciences and Engineering Research Council (NSERC) of Canada and Conselho Nacional de Desenvolvimento Científico e Tecnologico (CNPq) of Brazil; Social Sciences and Humanities Research Council (SSHRC) of Canada; University of British Columbia (UBC) President's fellowship to one of us (A.W.D.); Dr. Wagner Rossi, Deputado do Estado de Sao Paulo; Mayor of Nuporanga; Dr. F.A.M. Duarte and staff of the University of Sao Paulo (USP) Computer Center, Virginia Green of the UBC Faculty of Arts Computing Center; Yom Tov Shamash of UBC for translating questionnaires into Portuguese; Lina Azoubel of USP for pretesting questionnaires; Drs. N.E. Schwartz and N.E. Waxler Morrison of UBC for helpful comments and suggestions; Jose, Pia, Maura, and Elsa of Nuporanga; and all the residents of Vila Diogo for their consent and cooperation in this project.

References

Al-Isi, I.J.; Kanawati, A.A.; McLaren, D.S.: Formal education of mothers and their nutritional behavior. J. Nutr. Educ. *7:* 22–24 (1975).

Anderson, M.A.; Austin, J.E.; Wray, J.D.; Zeitlin, M.F.: Supplementary feeding; in Austin, Zeitlin, Nutrition intervention in developing countries – an overview, pp. 25–48 (Oelgeschlager, Gunn & Hain, Cambridge 1981).

Angeleli, W.A.; Vichi, F.L.; Vannucchi, H.; Desai, I.D.; Dutra de Oliveira, J.E.: Dietary supplementation and improvement in physical work performance of agricultural migrant workers of southern Brazil. Arch. Latinoam. Nutr. *33:* 159–169 (1983).

Anonymous: An action-oriented research, development and training programme in nutrition. WHO Chron. *33:* 225–227 (1979).

Antonov, A.N.: Children born during the siege of Leningrad in 1942. J. Pediat. *30:* 250–259 (1947).

Avioli, L.: Calcium and phosphorus; in Goodhart, Shils, Modern nutrition in health and disease; 6th ed., pp. 294–309 (Lea & Febiger, Philadelphia 1980).

Basta, S.S.: Nutrition and health in low income urban areas of the third world. Ecol. Food Nutr. *6:* 113–124 (1977).

Beaton, G.H.: Evaluation of nutrient intake: new statistical approaches. Arch. Latinoam. Nutr. *25:* 31–46 (1975).

Beaton, G.H.; Patwardhan, V.N.: Physiological and practical considerations of nutrient function and requirements. Annex 1; in Beaton, Bengoa, Nutrition in preventive medicine, pp. 445–482 (WHO, Genève 1976).

Beutler, E.: Iron; in Goodhart, Shils, Modern nutrition in health and disease; 6th ed., pp. 324–354 (Lea & Febiger, Philadelphia 1980).

Burk, M.C.; Pao, E.M.: Analysis of food consumption survey data for developing countries (FAO, Roma 1980).

Church, M.; Doughty, J.: Value of traditional food practices in nutrition education. J. hum. Nutr. *30:* 9–12 (1976).

Committee on Food Consumption Patterns: Assessing changing food consumption patterns (National Academy Press, Washington 1981).

Daly, J.A.; Davis, J.H.; Robertson, R.: Determinants of health and nutritional status; in Klein, Read, Riecken, Brown, Pradilla, Daza, Evaluating the impact of nutrition and health problems, pp. 7–34 (Plenum Press, New York 1979).

Desai, I.D.; Garcia Tavares, M.L.; Dutra de Oliveira, B.S.; Desai, M.I.; Cevallos Romero, L.S.; Vichi, F.L.; Duarte, F.A.M.; Dutra de Oliveira, J.E.: Anthropometric and cycloergometric assessment of the nutritional status of the children of agricultural migrant workers in southern Brazil. Am. J. clin. Nutr. *34:* 1925–1934 (1981).

Desai, I.D.; Garcia Tavares, M.L.; Dutra de Oliveira, B.S.; Douglas, A.; Duarte, F.A.M.; Dutra de Oliveira, J.E.: Food habits and nutritional status of agricultural migrant workers in southern Brazil. Am. J. clin. Nutr. *33:* 702–714 (1980).

Dickenson, J.P.: Brazil (Dawson & Sons, London 1978).

Dorea, J.G.; Almeida, I.S.; Queiroz, E.F.O.; Horner, M.R.: Nutritional status and zinc nutriture in infants and children in a poor urban community of Brazil. Ecol. Food Nutr. *12:* 1–6 (1982).

Drummond, T.: Using the method of Paulo Freire in nutrition education: an experimental plan for community action in northeast Brazil. Cornell Int. Nutr. Monogr. Ser., No. 3, pp. 17–46 (Cornell University, Ithaca 1975).

Filho, M.B.; Lucena, M.A.F. de; Coelho, H.A.L.: Protein-calorie malnutrition in three Brazilian state capitals: Sao Luis, Recife, and Sao Paulo. Bull. Pan Am. Health Org. *15:* 231–240 (1981).

Fomon, S.J.: Normal growth, failure to thrive and obesity; in Fomon, Infant nutrition; 2nd ed., pp. 34–94 (Saunders, Philadelphia 1974).

Francois, P.; Sizaret, F.: Pulse consumption in Brazil – protein intake threatened by uncertain supply. Food Nutr. *7:* 11–17 (1981).

Freire, P.: Pedagogy of the oppressed, pp. 57–75 (Continuum Publishing, New York 1981).

Frisancho, A.R.: Triceps skin fold and upper arm muscle size norms for assessment of nutritional status. Am. J. clin. Nutr. *27:* 1052–1058 (1974).

Ghosh, S.; Manmohan; Yayathi, T.: Domestic visualisation: an innovative approach to nutrition education. Environ. Child Health *23:* 282–285 (1977).

Gussow, J.D.; Contento, I.: Nutrition education in a changing world. A conceptualization and selective review; in Bourne, Wld Rev. Nutr. Diet., vol. 44, pp. 1–57 (Karger, Basel 1984).

Harper, A.E.: Some comments on protein and amino acid utilization. Am. J. clin. Nutr. *11:* 382–388 (1982).

Harwood, A.: The hot-cold theory of disease. J. Am. med. Ass. *216:* 1153–1158 (1971).

Health and Welfare Canada: Recommended nutrient intakes for Canadians (Canadian Government Publishing Centre, Ottawa 1983).

Hennigan, K.M.; Flay, B.R.; Haag, R.A.: Clarification of concepts and terms commonly used in evaluative research; in Klein, Read, Riecken, Brown, Pradilla, Daza, Evaluating the impact of nutrition and health programs, pp. 387–423 (Plenum Press, New York 1979).

Hewlett, S.A.: The cruel dilemmas of development: twentieth-century Brazil (Basic Books, New York 1980).

Huffman, S.L.: Child spacing: for maternal and child health. Mothers and children. Bull. Infant Feed. maternal Nutr. *4:* 1–2 (1984).

Interdepartmental Committee for National Development: Nutrition survey: northeast Brazil, March-May 1963 (US Government Printing Office, Washington 1965).

Iyengar, L.: Influence of diet on the outcome of pregnancy in Indian women; in Chavez, Bourges, Basta, Prognosis for the undernourished surviving child, vol. 2, pp. 53–59 (Karger, Basel 1975).

Jansen, J.R.; Jansen, N.B.; Shigetomi, C.T.; Harper, J.M.: Effect of income and geographic region on the nutritional value of diets in Brazil. Am. J. clin. Nutr. *30:* 955–964 (1977).

Jelliffe, D.B.: The assessment of the nutritional status of the community. WHO Monogr. Ser., No. 53 (WHO, Genève 1966).

King, M.H.; King, K.M.; Morley, D.C.; Burgess, H.J.L.; Burgess, A.P.: Nutrition for developing countries (Oxford University Press, London 1972).

Kluck, P.A.: The society and its environment; in Nyrop, Brazil – a country study; 4th ed., pp. 81–157 (US Government Printing Office, Washington 1983).

Knight, P.T.; Moran, R.: Brazil – human resources special report (World Bank, Washington 1979).

Kolasa, K.M.: Nutrition education and changing behavior; in Harper, Davis, Nutrition in the 1980s: constraints on our knowledge, pp. 415–422 (Liss, New York 1981).

Marcondes, E.; Berquo, E.S.; Yunes, J.; Luongo, J.; Souza Martins, J. de; Zacchi, M.A.S.; Levy, M.S.F.; Hegg, R.: Estudo antropométrico de crianças Brasileiras de zero a doze anos de idade. Anais Nestlé, Fasciculo No. 84 (1971).
Molony, C.H.: Systematic valence coding of Mexican 'hot'-'cold' food. Ecol. Food. Nutr. *4:* 67–74 (1975).
Murphy, R.S.; Michael, G.A.: Methodologic considerations of the National Health and Nutrition Examination Survey. Am. J. clin. Nutr. *35:* suppl., pp. 1225–1258 (1981).
National Center for Health Statistics (NCHS): Data collected in its Health Examination Surveys; in Nelson, Text book of pediatrics, pp. 37–39 (Saunders, Philadelphia 1979).
Nyrop, R.F.: Brazil – a country study; 4th ed., pp. xiii–xviii, xxi–xxix (US Government Printing Office, Washington 1983).
Patrick, G.F.; Simoes, M.H.R.: Least-cost diets in Cristalina, Goias, Brazil. Arch. Latinoam. Nutr. *21:* 371–380 (1971).
Pollitt, E.: Child poverty in South America: reflections in its magnitude, and the basic-need development approach. Arch. Latinoam. Nutr. *31:* 235–249 (1981).
Praun, A.: Nutrition education: development or alienation? Hum. Nutr. appl. Nutr. *36A:* 28–34 (1982).
Richardson, B.D.: Malnutrition and nutritional anthropometry. J. trop. Pediat. *26:* 80–84 (1980).
Robinson, C.H.: Basic nutrition and diet therapy; 4th ed. (Macmillan, New York 1980).
Roett, R.: Brazil – politics in a patrimonial society (Praeger, New York 1978).
Sanjur, D.: Social and cultural perspectives in nutrition (Prentice-Hall, Englewood Cliffs 1982).
Schmidt, B.J.; Feitosa, D.H.; Funari, S.A.; Ribeiro, A.C.; Thomas, C.J.; Oliveira, J.A.; Motta, Y.; Takahashi, N.; Miranda, J.E.G.B.; Bagatin, E.: Breast-feeding in Sorocaba, S. Paulo, Brasil. Study performed on mothers belonging to different socio-economic levels (English abstr.). Courrier *30:* 561–567 (1980).
Scrimshaw, N.S.: Significance of the appraisal of the nutrient intake and the nutritional status of man. Am. J. clin. Nutr. *11:* 331–334 (1962).
Scrimshaw, N.S.; Lockwood, R.: Interpretation of data on human food availability and nutrient consumption. Food Nutr. Bull. *2:* 29–38 (1980).
Shrimpton, R.: Nutrition and development in Brasil; MSc thesis, London (1975).
Sousa, P.L.R.; Barros, F.C.; Pinheiro, G.N.M.; Gazalle, R.V.: Patterns of weaning in south Brazil. J. trop. pediat. environ. Health *21:* 210–211 (1975).
Swann, M.A.: Nutritional assessment of agricultural migrant workers in southern Brazil; MSc thesis, Vancouver (1979).
Synderman, S.E.: Nutrition in infancy and adolescence; in Goodhart, Shils, Modern nutrition in health and disease; 6th ed., pp. 753–780 (Lea & Febiger, Philadelphia 1980).
Thomas, V.: Differences in income, nutrition and poverty within Brazil. World Bank Staff Working Paper, No. 505 (World Bank, Washington 1982).
Thomson, A.M.; Billewicz, W.Z.; Thompson, B.; McGregor, I.A.: Body weight changes during pregnancy and lactation in rural African (Gambian) women. J. Obstet. Gynaec. Br. Commonw. *73:* 724–733 (1966).

Tragler, A.T.; Bhatt, S.S.; Fernandez, A.: Assessment of health education in nutrition. J. trop. Pediat. *27:* 221–223 (1981).
Waddell, C.: The nutritional status and physical work performance of children of migrant agricultural workers in southern Brazil; MSc thesis, Vancouver (1981).
Ward, J.O.; Amoni, D.: Diets of urban migrants in northeast Brazil: an economic analysis. Nutr. Rep. int. *21:* 11–24 (1980).
Weil, T.E.; Black, J.K.; Blutstein, H.I.; Johnston, K.T.; McMorris, D.S.: Area handbook for Brazil; 3rd ed. (US Government Printing Office, Washington 1975).
Wishik, S.M.; Stern, R.G.: Impact of birth spacing on maternal and child nutrition, conceptualization of research approaches; in Chavez, Bourges, Basta, Proc 9th Int. Congr. of Nutrition, Prognosis for the Undernourished Surviving Child, vol. 2, pp. 32–36 (Karger, Basel 1972).
Wolgemuth, J.C.; Latham, M.C.; Hall, A.; Chesher, A.; Crompton, D.W.T.: Worker productivity and the nutritional status of Kenyan road construction laborers. Am. J. clin. Nutr. *36:* 68–78 (1982).
World Health Organization: Contemporary patterns of breast-feeding (WHO, Genève 1981a).
World Health Organization: Guidelines for training community health workers in nutrition. WHO Publ., No. 59 (WHO, Genève 1981b).
Wright, M.G.M.; Horner, M.R.; Charini, L.H.: Approaches for increasing soybean use by low-income Brazilian families. J. Nutr. Educ. *14:* 105–107 (1982).

Prof. I.D. Desai, PhD, The University of British Columbia, School of Family and Nutritional Sciences, 2205 East Mall, Vancouver, B.C., V6T 1W5 (Canada)

Bourne GH (ed): Aspects of Food Production, Consumption and Energy Values.
World Rev Nutr Diet. Basel, Karger, 1990, vol 61, pp 132–172

Nutritional Energetics in Fish: Energy and Protein Utilization in Rainbow Trout *(Salmo gairdneri)*

C.Y. Cho, S.J. Kaushik

Fisheries Branch, Ontario Ministry of Natural Resources and Department of Nutritional Sciences, University of Guelph, Guelph, Ont., Canada;
Laboratoire de Nutrition et d'Elevage des Poissons INRA, St-Pée-sur-Nivelle, Ascain, France

Contents

Introduction

Nutritional Energetics

Nutritional energetics, or bioenergetics, is the study of the balance between supply of dietary fuels, expenditure and storage gain, and requires an examination of the physiological processes by which energy is quantitatively transformed within a living organism. However, nutritional energetics usually concentrates upon the prediction of how the energy demands of the whole animal are met by 'energy-yielding' nutrients from different diets. An understanding of the nutritional energetics of any productive animal is a first step to provide a defined and adequately balanced dietary regime, under any particular environment and to improve the efficiency of diet utilization.

Nutritionists deal with defined chemical entities which play a role in the animal either as tissue components and their precursors, or as fuels which upon catabolism lead to the formation of useful intermediates to permit the completion of energy-requiring processes. The completion of these processes results in either an increase in the energy content of the animal as a whole or in the release of heat. Thus the utilization of dietary fuels does not cause any change in the energy content of the whole system (the animal, its feed, or its surroundings). What gets changed is the form of the energy: the chemical energy of the diet gets wholly or partially converted to heat. The heat energy is less useful than the chemical energy of the diet, and this change is described by the increase in the entropy of the system. Schroedinger [1944] summarizes this by stating that 'animals consume negative entropy'. Thus animals do have a requirement for fuels which can be expressed as their energy equivalents, or even as an energy requirement.

Energy Requirements of Animals

Life exists in a thermodynamically unstable state and its continuation is dependent on the balance between dietary supply of fuels and heat production as a consequence of life-maintaining processes. In fact, if the dietary fuel supply is less than what is needed to sustain life processes and to support its voluntary activities, body tissues will be catabolized in addition to the dietary nutrients.

In additon, animals also need energy to grow, and to reproduce. Physical activity and thermoregulation also increase energy requirement. The animal's energy needs are influenced by the stage of the life cycle, by the season and by the environment. Young growing animals require more energy per unit of body weight for maintenance than mature animals, although reproductive activity increases the energy needs of mature animals. Environmental temperature plays an obvious role in influencing the fuel required to maintain body temperature in homeotherms but has an even greater influence in poikilotherms, such as fish, in which the rate of metabolism can change manyfold in response to changes in water temperature.

A full definition of the energy and nutrient requirements demands a knowledge of the partition of the dietary 'energy-yielding' components between catabolism as fuels and anabolism as in tissue. Measurements of these losses and gains involve the use of whole animals since this aspect of assessing nutritive value of a diet is a biological evaluation rather than a chemical or physical one.

Dietary Fuel Supply and Utilization

Both the quantity and quality of the diet influence the metabolic partition of the components between storage and catabolism as fuels. It is this flexibility on the part of the animal to use all three components of the diet as fuels which leads to the complexities of the interactions among proteins, lipids and carbohydrates. As a consequence, the energy value of the diet to

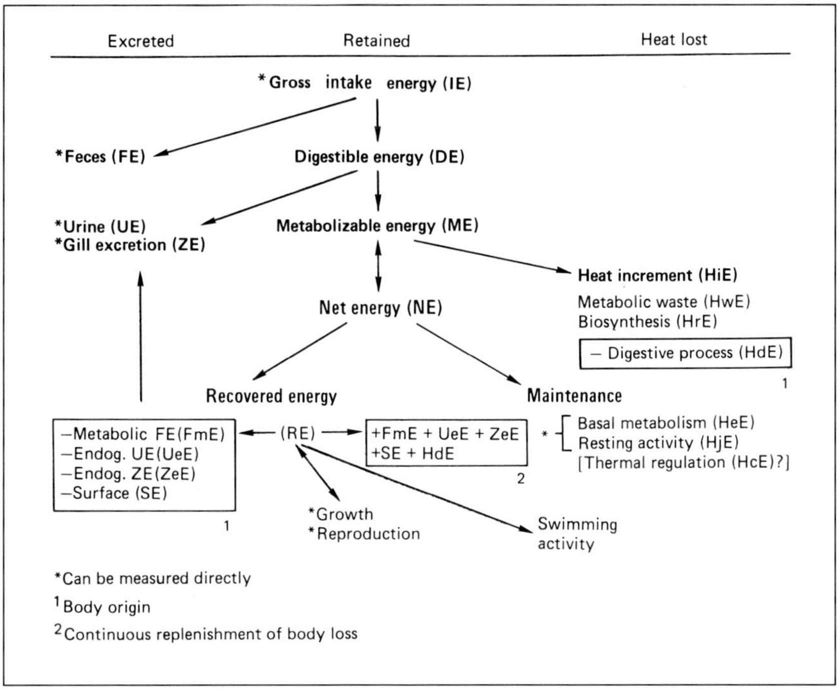

Fig. 1. Schematic presentation of the fate of dietary energy for fish categorizing the losses of energy which occur as feed is digested, and metabolized leaving a fraction of the dietary energy to be retained as new tissue. From Cho et al. [1982].

the animal must be defined before drawing any conclusions as to the effect of the diet upon the growth of the animal.

Dietary intake energy from the absorbed nutrients involves a multiplicity of physiological processes for their utilization. Any model to describe such a system will necessarily be elaborate if it is to interrelate the losses which occur in the utilization of dietary fuel for tissue growth. Such a scheme is shown in figure 1 and a glossary of the terminology is provided by NRC-NAC [1981a].

Specificities of Fish Nutritional Energetics

In the area of fish nutrition, an understanding of protein utilization is of special significance. It is well established that more of the energy requirement of fish is met from protein and lipid than is the case in omnivores, birds and mammals. This is possibly because most fishes may have more obligate need for amino acids and fatty acids as an energy source than other animals. The dependence of carnivorous fish on a high protein diet derives not only from a highly developed capacity to metabolize protein [Smith et al., 1978a, b] but also from a limited ability to digest and catabolize carbohydrates [Cowey and Luquet, 1983].

Availability of Dietary Fuel

Energy is not a nutrient but a property of the 'energy-yielding' nutrients when they are oxidized and metabolized. All organic compounds in fish diet release heat upon combustion, and thus are potential sources of energy. However, most dietary carbohydrates, such as raw starch from plant feed ingredients, are little digested by carnivorous fish such as salmonids, and their use as energy sources in the diet formulations is of little practical significance. Lipids and proteins, therefore, provide the primary sources of dietary fuels. Physiologically, proteins and lipids form a major part of a structure of a fish, but the need for energy can preclude their incorporation into tissues and lead to their catabolism.

The gross energy value of the diet depends upon its chemical composition, and the mean values of heats of combustion of carbohydrate, protein and lipid being: 17.2, 23.6 and 39.5 kJ/g respectively [Brafield and Llewellyn, 1982]. However, the inherent chemical makeup of the diet influences only its heat of combustion or gross energy and the total amount of the nutrients in a diet. This yields no information on whether or not the nutrients are 'available' to fish through the digestive process.

Importance of Digestibility Measurements

Ingested dietary nutrients such as protein, lipid and carbohydrate in diets must be hydrolyzed prior to utilization by the fish. Digested protein, lipid and carbohydrate provide such essential nutrients as amino acids, fatty acids and glucose and also fulfill a major dietary function in supplying digestible energy (DE) to fuel metabolic activity. Dietary protein and lipid are both 'tissue-yielding' and 'energy-yielding' nutrients and the digestibilities determine the 'potentially available' amount of tissue components and energy for utilization by the animal.

Prior to any attempt to formulate diets for fish, it is then necessary to determine ingredient digestibilities as the digestibility coefficients of the nutrients in the individual dietary ingredients determine the availability of energy and nutrients in the diets. In the context of fish nutrition, digestibility coefficients are little affected by biotic and abiotic factors and these coefficient values of individual ingredients are additive [Cho and Kaushik, 1985], so that the final content of DE and nutrients in the diets can be predicted from the digestibility coefficients and levels of inclusion of the ingredients in the diet.

Methods to Measure Apparent Digestibility Coefficients of Feed Ingredients

In the aquatic environment, as both feed and fecal particles are transited through the same medium, to separate feces from water and to avoid contamination of the feces by uneaten feed, it has been necessary to resort to the use of approaches other than those used to measure digestibilities with mammals and birds.

Nose [1960] collected samples of rectal contents by gently squeezing out the fecal material from the rectum. Windell et al. [1978] obtained samples of rectal contents by applying suction to the anus or by dissecting the fish. These techniques involved handling the fish and exposing them to considerable stress. Forced evacuation and disection of the rectum could result in the addition of physiological fluids and intestinal epithelium to the rectal contents. Smith [1971] confined the fish in metabolic chambers and collected the feces that were voided naturally into the water. Ogino et al. [1973] collected the feces by passing the effluent water from the fish tanks through a filtration column which is effective, but more suitable for smaller quantity of feces collection. Choubert et al. [1979] used a system consisting of mechanically rotating screens to filter out fecal material which avoids any physiological stress and allows collection over long periods, but requires considerable maintenance to operate.

To avoid stress to fish and to simplify feces collection, a digestibility system was developed (fig. 2) to allow the separation of feces by sedimentation for routine measurements of digestibility of feed ingredients or compound diets during growth experiments.

Comparison of Different Methods

Table 1 shows comparison of results on apparent digestibility coefficient (ADC) obtained using different methods. The studies all included herring fish meal although the different studies used different samples. The

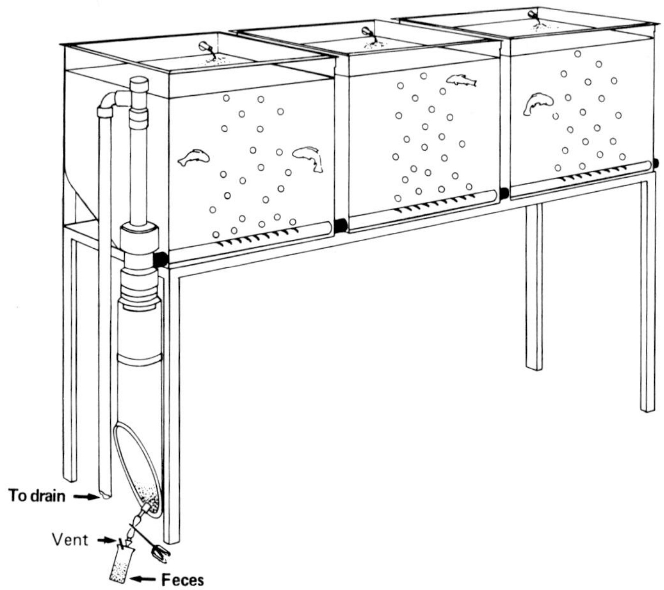

Fig. 2. Fish digestibility system consisting of 3 fiberglass tanks with common drain-pipe to feces settling column for the determination of digestibility coefficients of feed ingredients. A cooling jacket or ice bucket can be fitted around the settling column to preserve feces samples.

crude protein content of all the samples except that used by Smith et al. [1980] were very similar. The results for five of the studies allows calculation of the digestibility of the dry matter of the diets to give an indication of their overall digestibilities. 'Break-up or handling' loss of the feces as in the case of trough-netting, for instance, can lead to overestimation of the digestibility coefficients. Contamination of feces with endogenous material, principally nitrogenous compounds and lipid, while stripping the fish to remove the rectal contents, can lead to some underestimation.

Table 1. Apparent digestibility coefficients of herring meal determined with rainbow trout in different laboratories

Feces collection method[1]	Crude protein in herring meal, %	Digestibility coefficient, % mean		
		dry matter	crude protein	lipid
1 Metabolism chamber	75.8	–	86.7	–
2 Intestinal dissection	67.9	80.3	90.2	96.7
3 Anal suction	67.9	79.1	90.4	97.4
4 Trough-netting	67.9	84.4	94.6	96.8
5 Stripping	67.9	73.3	77.5	62.2
6 Stripping (personal data)	66.7	–	88.2	–
7 Guelph system	66.7	80.2	91.0	97.3

[1] (1) Smith et al. [1980]; (2–5) Windell et al. [1978].

Need for the Use of a Reference Diet

Very few potentially useful feed ingredients can be fed directly to an animal as the sole ingredient of a diet; it is always necessary to mix several ingredients to make an acceptable diet before feeding. Thus a determination of digestibility of a feed ingredient requires a comparison of the digestibilities of a reference diet and a test diet. The test should then be a mixture of the reference diet (70%) and the test ingredient (30%).

As quantitative collection of fish feces is difficult to achieve, the direct methods of digestibility measurements cannot be successfully used with fish. Edin [1918] introduced the use of chromic sesquioxide as digestion indicator to obviate the need to quantify dietary intake and feces output. Inclusion of this tracer in the diet allows the digestibility coefficients of the nutrients in the test diets to be calculated from measurements of the nutrient-to-indicator ratios in the diet and feces. Once these coefficients have been calculated for the reference and test diets, the corresponding digestibility coefficients can be calculated for the nutrients in the ingredient being tested.

The use of a reference diet assumes that there are no interactions among the components of the diet during digestion. Also adoption of this procedure allows the use of an adequately balanced diet with which to measure the digestibility of different feed ingredients. Inclusion of such a reference diet allows a measurement of normal feed intake and growth rate and also confirms the adequacy of the experimental diets.

ADC are then calculated using the following formulae:

ADC of reference or test diet (%) = [1 – (F/D × Dcr/Fcr)] × 100,

ADC of test feed ingredient (%) =

(ADC of test diet – 0.7 ADC of reference diet)/0.3,

where D = % nutrient or kJ energy in diet; F = % nutrient or kJ energy in feces; Dcr = % chromic sesquioxide in diet; Fcr = % chromic sesquioxide in feces.

ADC Values for Different Fish Feed Ingredients

Variation in the digestibility of diets is generally the major factor affecting their usefulness as energy and nutrient sources to the animal, since the fecal loss is the major loss of the ingesta. Therefore the digestible energy values and the digestibilities of individual nutrients (protein, lipid and carbohydrate) should be used to estimate levels of available energy and nutrients in the feed ingredients for the formulation of diets.

The commercially available diets used in fish culture today result in the loss to the fish of between 20 and 40% of the intake in the feces. There are some feed ingredients in which as much as 50–80% of the dietary energy is lost as feces. Fish, particularly salmonids, digest protein and lipid very well (table 2) and simple sugars such as monosaccharides and hydrolyzed or gelatinized starch are also well-digested by rainbow trout. However, raw starch is poorly digested by rainbow trout and thus the DE value of some raw starch should be assessed at as little as 4 MJ DE/kg in calculations to predict the energy value of formulated diets. Some grain by-products such as ground corn and wheat middlings are included mainly as a 'binder and filler' to enhance the durability of the pelleted feeds. Clearly the appropriate level at which to include these poorly digested materials represents a compromise between the nutritional value of the diet and practical considerations such as the mechanical durability of the feed aggregate.

Digestible Energy Values

Table 2 lists the digestible energy values determined for a number of different feed ingredients using rainbow trout. The DE values approach the gross energy values for the high protein materials such as spray-dried blood meal, herring meal, cooked full-fat soybeans and soybean protein concentrate, indicating a high degree of digestion and absorption. However, for the feed ingredients which contain a substantial level of carbohydrate, such

Table 2. ADC and DE values of ingredients measured with rainbow trout[1]

Ingredient name	International feed no.	Digestibility coefficient				DE MJ/kg
		DM, %	CP, %	lipid, %	GE, %	
Alfalfa meal	1–00–023	39	87	71	43	7.7
Blood meal, animal						
Spray-dried	5–00–381	91	99	–	89	19.4
Flame-dried	5–00–381	55	16	–	50	10.9
Brewer's dried yeast	7–05–527	76	91	–	77	13.9
Corn, yellow	4–02–935	23	95	–	39	6.6
Corn gluten feed	5–02–903	23	92	–	29	5.4
Corn gluten meal	5–09–318	80	96	–	83	17.6
Corn dist. dried sol.	5–02–844	46	85	71	51	10.7
Feather meal, poultry	5–03–795	75	58	–	70	15.7
Fish meal, herring	5–02–000	85	92	97	91	18.8
Meat and bone meal	5–09–321	78	85	73	85	15.0
Poultry byprod. meal	5–03–798	52	68	79	71	13.9
Rapeseed meal	5–03–871	35	77	–	45	8.1
Soybean, fullfat, cook.	5–04–597	78	96	94	85	19.0
Soybean meal, dehull.	5–04–612	74	96	–	75	13.5
Wheat middlings	4–05–205	35	92	–	46	7.6
Whey, dehydrated	4–01–182	97	96	–	94	13.4
Starch, raw		37	–	–	49	8.6
Starch, gelatinized		86	–	–	86	13.3
Fish protein concentrate		90	95	–	94	17.2
Soybean protein concentrate		77	97	–	84	15.4
C202-Guelph Reference diet		75	94	95	80	16.5

[1] All values are cumulative averages of compiled data. DM = Dry matter; CP = crude protein; GE = gross energy; DE = digestible energy; 1 MJ = 239 kcal.

as yellow corn, corn gluten feed and rapeseed meal, the DE values are less than half of the gross energy values, confirming that starch and fiber are poorly digested by rainbow trout. The DE values of the feed ingredients are also closely correlated with the dry matter digestibilities.

Considering possible factors that might affect the ADC of dietary ingredients, it has been well established that neither environmental factors like temperature or salinity nor biotic factors like age have significant influence on the digestibility of nutrients. Only two major factors will be dealt with on detail here.

Water Temperature and ADC

In response to an increase in temperature, the primary response of fish is to increase their feed intake. They also increase their metabolic rates and one of the constant features is the increase in the rate of transit of ingesta through the digestive tract with increasing water temperature [Fange and Grove, 1979], and this may affect the digestibility of the diet. On the other hand, the longer gastric evacuation time may compensate for a less efficient digestive process at the lower water temperatures [Fauconneau et al., 1983].

A number of works has been undertaken with rainbow trout to study the effect of different temperatures on digestibility [Cho, 1987; Kaushik, 1981]. Results of one such study conducted at Guelph are reported in table 3. These results confirm the observations of other authors and show that ADC of dry matter, crude protein, lipid and gross energy are not significantly influenced by the water temperature.

If one considers the apparent digestibility of the oils and fats which are one of the major fuel sources, the results from another experiment (table 4) indicate that the ADC of the practical diet and oils were not influenced by the range of water temperatures employed in these studies. The fish oil and plant oils (rapeseed, soybean and linseed) were well digested (ADC = 80–95%) at all 3 water temperatures. However, the ADC of lard and tallow were affected by the water temperature (70–78 and 58–66%, respectively) and lower than that of oils. A definite interaction between the melting point of the lipid employed and water temperature is observed. The ADC of lard and tallow are clearly poorer at lower water temperatures, in contrast with the lack of effect of water temperatures on the lower melting

Table 3. Effect of water temperature on the ADC of a practical reference diet in rainbow trout

	Water temperature, °C				Mean
	9	12	15	18	
Dry matter, %	69	69	68	70	69
Crude protein, %	93	91	91	94	92
Lipid, %	91	89	90	93	91
Gross energy, %	76	76	75	78	76

point oils. This confirms that lard and tallow should be avoided as a source of lipid in diets which are designed for fish culture in cold waters (e.g. below 10 °C).

Feeding Level and ADC

Any change in the feeding levels due to changes in water temperature, or to other husbandry practices, may alter the amount of total digested and absorbed energy and nutrients from feed consumed. However, it has been demonstrated that neither the frequency of feeding nor the level of feed intake affect the ADC of dry matter, crude protein, lipid and gross energy (table 5).

Table 4. Percent ADC of oils and fats at different water temperatures in rainbow trout

Oils and fats	Low/high melting point °C	Water temperatures 5 °C	10 °C	15 °C
Fish oil		80	81	81
Rapeseed oil	0/–12[1]	85	89	90
Soybean oil	–7/–8	92	93	91
Linseed oil	–18/–27[1]	92	95	95
Lard	28/48	70	76	78
Tallow	45/48	58	64	66

[1] Coagulation point.

Table 5. ADC of the practical diet at different feeding levels in rainbow trout

Feeding levels, %	100[1]	80	60	40	Mean
Feed intake/day, g/kg BW[2]	15	12	9	6	
Dry matter, %	69	65	66	70	67
Crude protein, %	91	90	91	92	91
Lipid, %	92	92	92	94	93
Gross energy, %	75	74	76	78	76

[1] Full feeding – fish were fed 3 times a day to satiety at 15 °C water temperature.
[2] Fish BW = 50–100 g/fish.

In understanding of these values of DE and nutrients, it is emphasized that the digestibility coefficients are only an indication of the potential contribution of the energy and nutrients from the ingredient. These values do not serve as measures of the 'utilizable' energy nor of the productivity of the diet.

Metabolizable Energy

Definition of Metabolizable Energy

Digestion of a diet leads to the absorption of amino acids, fatty acids and sugars which are the principal metabolic fuels for the body. Catabolism of lipid and carbohydrate results in the formation of carbon dioxide and water, the fully oxidized products of carbon and hydrogen, respectively. However, the catabolism of amino acids yields ammonia, in addition to carbon dioxide and water. These nonfecal losses, of which ammonia amounts to about 85%, are excreted via two organs: gills and kidneys. These energy losses, mainly through the gills (branchial energy loss, ZE) and some through in the kidneys (urinary N loss, UE), are unaccounted for by the DE value of a diet. The physiologically utilizable fuel value of the diet to the fish is the metabolizable energy (ME) and is defined as follows:

$$ME = DE - (ZE + UE) \text{ (fig. 1).}$$

There are few interactions of any significance between feed ingredients in diets which might influence their utilization at the digestion level. Thus, whereas the DE value of a feed is relatively independent of the composition of the diet on which it is fed and the contribution of DE from individual feed ingredients to the total diet are additive, in contrast, the loss of combustible matter through the gills and in the urine depends upon the biological value of the total protein and its amount in relation to DE in the diet. This ratio of dietary digestible protein to DE is in turn influenced by the proportions of the different feed ingredients included in the diet. Consequently, the contribution of a given feed ingredient to the ME of a diet is dependent on the composition of the diet, since it is the overall balance of the amino acids and energy in the diet which influences the retention of protein by the body and hence governs the metabolic loss of nitrogenous end products.

Validity of ME Values

There is much controversy amongst fish nutritionists as to the relative usefulness of DE and ME values as a means of comparing the fuel values to the fish of different feed ingredients for diet formulations [Smith, 1971; Cho et al., 1982]. The success with poultry has led to the extrapolation of poultry ME values to compare feeds for other species, even fish. ME values have been chosen by poultry nutritionists for a practical reason that birds void feces and urine together. These values have been used for the last two decades as a basis for the prediction of the effects upon 'productivity' of changing dietary formulations. Measurement of ME values of diets is simple in poultry. In mammals, pigs for example, the measurement of ME requires the separate collection and analysis of urine.

For most diets formulated to contain balanced protein and energy levels for the pig, there is a constant relationship between the DE and ME values [Diggs et al., 1965], ME equalling 96% of DE. Thus, even in the case of mammals, the extra experimental work involved in determining ME does not appear to be warranted. In the case of fish, the ME values expressed as a fraction of the DE values ranged from 0.72 to 0.93 (mean = 0.87) [NRC-NAS, 1981b]. This shows that for most diets, a much higher proportion of the absorption of the absorbed dietary energy is excreted through the gills and kidneys than was excreted in the urine by the pig.

It is usual to feed pigs with diets containing from 13 to 18% protein, which is much lower than the protein levels of 35–50% which are common in the diets fed to salmonid fish. Thus, a larger amount of the energy intake of fish is provided as nitrogenous compounds which lead to the excretion of correspondingly larger amounts of ammonia. An additional factor contributing to the larger difference between ME and DE values for rainbow trout [Smith et al., 1980] could be the procedures employed to separate and collect nitrogen excreted via the gills and kidneys which possibly lead to a negative nitrogen balance.

Thus, fish nutritionists who must ascribe fuel values to different ingredients to formulate balanced diets should employ DE values and avoid ME values obtained by methods that may be susceptible to gross error as indicated by excessive nitrogen losses or other signs of disturbed protein metabolism.

It is recognized that theoretically, ME is the more appropriate measure of utilizable fuel value in evaluating compound diets. Accurate measurement of nitrogen loss through the gills is very important to quantify

ME in diets. However, obtaining reliable ME values is dependent on the development of techniques to measure the nonfecal losses.

Measurement of Metabolic Losses

Determination of the ME values of diets for fish is technically difficult because of the need to quantify both gill and urinary losses. Smith [1971] attempted to overcome these difficulties and developed a procedure which allowed the estimation of the ME values of a number of feed ingredients and diets using rainbow trout. Before the assays, the fish were inserted with a cannula for urine collection. The fish were then confined in a metabolism chamber with a diaphragm separating the front from the rear portion of the body, and they were force-fed under anesthesia, the feed being tested as a single daily meal.

Brett and Zala [1975] determined the diurnal pattern of nitrogen excretion of young sockeye salmon *(Oncorhynchus nerka)* by allowing ammonia to build up during alternate periodical closed-circuit cycles. Kaushik [1980] and his co-workers have estimated the post-prandial excretion rates by continuous measurement in a flow-through system connected to an autoanalyzer. This method allows continuous monitoring of ammonia and urea nitrogen excretion under physiological conditions and they have measured nitrogen excretion even in larval fish [Kaushik et al., 1982]. Under these conditions, however, attention should be paid to the maintenance of a constant flow rate and a precise measurement of low concentrations of ammonia in the outlet water.

Energy Equivalents of Nitrogenous Excreta

The energy value of ammonia was reported to be 90.6 kcal/mol by Needham [1931], 82 kcal/mol by Brody [1945] and 90 kcal/mol by Pilgrim [1954]. However, Elliott and Davison [1975] calculated from the heats of formation that the energy value of ammonia, more correctly the specific enthalpy of combustion of ammonia, was 83.2 kcal/mol or 20.5 kJ/g, which is identical to the value by Brafield and Llewellyn [1982]. The energy value of urea in the aqueous state is 154.4 kcal/mol or 10.8 kJ/g. The energy values of excreted ammonia and urea given by Elliott and Davison are equivalent to 24.9 and 23.1 kJ/g nitrogen, respectively. Since the major part of the nitrogen ($>85\%$) is excreted as ammonia, it is reasonable to use the value of 24.9 kJ/g N estimate the energy loss of the nonfecal nitrogen excretion.

Indirect Estimation of ME

As these direct measurements of nonfecal nitrogen losses which allow either ammonia to build up to a measurable concentration or which require sophisticated equipment are neither satisfactory, nor practical for routine application, it is advisable to use indirect methods to estimate branchial and urinary losses of nitrogen [Cho and Kaushik, 1985].

Losses of digested, absorbed nitrogen occur mainly through the gills and in the urine with a negligible amount from surface losses such as mucous and scales. Therefore, total nonfecal nitrogen loss, branchial and urinary, is estimated by the difference between digested nitrogen and recovered nitrogen as shown in the following expression:

$$ZN + UN = DN - RN,$$
$$ZE + UE = (ZN + UN) \times 24.9 \text{ kJ/g N},$$
$$ME = DE - (ZE + UE),$$

where ZN = branchial N loss; UN = urinary N loss; DN = digestible N intake; RN = recovered tissue N; ZE = branchial energy loss; UE = urinary energy loss; ME = metabolizable energy; DE = digestible energy.

ME versus Dietary Protein: Energy Balance

The protein-sparing effects of fats and of pretreated starch have led to a new generation of fish diets with decreased levels of protein and increased levels of DE. The overall performance of fish with such diets has been well documented [Cho and Woodward, 1989]. Kaushik and Oliva-Teles [1985] showed recently that an increase in the dietary DE by an increase in dietary nonprotein energy led to a decrease in ammonia nitrogen excretion and hence to an increase in ME.

As illustrated in figure 3 the same lot of fish meal can be used in different rations which can be fed under different husbandry conditions. In the case of diet A, the protein from the fish meal is utilized to a minimum for energy purposes since the diet contains enough nonprotein 'energy-yielding' nutrient (lipid). Hence the reduced oxidation of protein and nonfecal nitrogen loss increase the ME value of the fish meal. But in the case of diet B, a high level of fish meal (protein) and with low energy (lipid) content in the diet increases the oxidation of protein to satisfy the energy needs of the fish and this leads to a higher oxidation of the protein and excretion of nonfecal nitrogen. Accordingly, the ME value of the fish meal is reduced because of the poor balance of protein/energy in the diet, even though the fish meal is the same as that used in diet A. This demonstrates

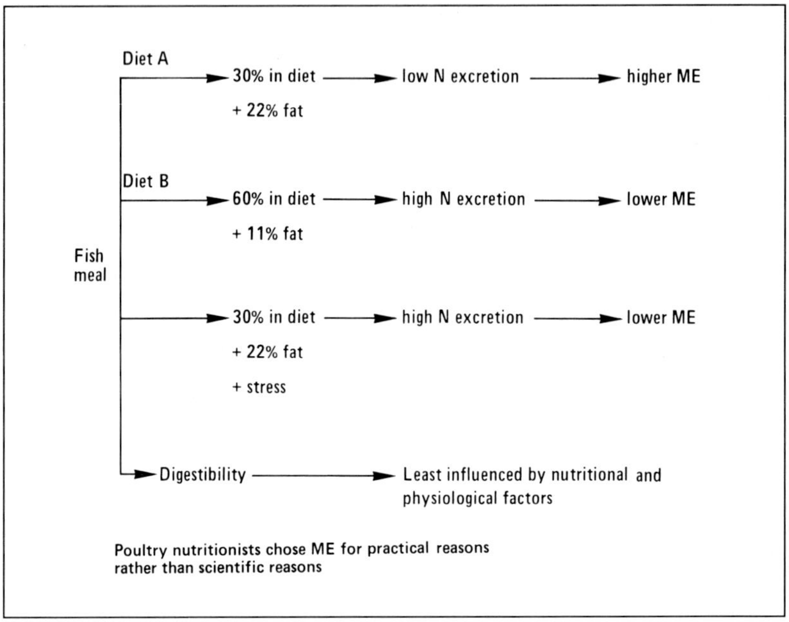

Fig. 3. Schematic illustration of the factors affecting ME value of fish meal.

that ME cannot be used for the evaluation of individual ingredients but should be used as a measure of the balance of protein and energy in fish diets. ME has significance only as long as it has been measured with respect to an animal's response to a complete diet in a given set of biological and environmental conditions.

The metabolic loss of nitrogen through excretion following the intake of different compound diets can be estimated by measuring nitrogen retained by the fish. This is simply digestible nitrogen intake minus nitrogen recovered over the experimental period determined through proximate analysis.

In table 6, nonfecal energy losses (ZE + UE) were calculated by multiplying 24.9 kJ/g N with nonfecal nitrogen losses (ZN + UN) [Cho and Watanabe, 1986]. No differences in nonfecal energy losses were observed at a given water temperature. The loss of nonfecal energy (branchial [ZE] + urinary [UE]), and total heat loss (HE) per kg feed intake were much greater at 7.5 °C than at other temperatures. This suggests that if the tem-

Table 6. Partition of dietary energy and energy retention efficiencies

Lipid %	Water temp. °C	MJ/kg feed intake					ERE
		DE	RE	ZE+UE	ME	HE	
13	7.5	15.0	5.1	0.9	14.1	9.0	0.34
	12.5	15.1	7.1	0.8	14.3	7.2	0.47
	17.5	15.6	7.6	0.8	14.8	7.6	0.46
18	7.5	16.7	6.3	0.9	15.8	9.5	0.38
	12.5	16.8	8.6	0.7	16.1	7.5	0.51
	17.5	16.9	8.5	0.8	16.1	7.6	0.50
23	7.5	17.2	5.9	0.9	16.3	10.4	0.34
	12.5	17.8	9.8	0.7	17.1	7.3	0.55
	17.5	17.9	9.1	0.8	17.1	8.0	0.50

RE (recovered energy) = GE in final carcass – GE in initial carcass. ZE + UE = 24.9 MJ (kg digest. N intake – kg recovered N). HE (total heat loss) = Heat increment of feeding + Fasing heat production = ME – RE. ERE (energy retention efficiency) = RE/DE.

perature declines much below optimum, the ability of fish to utilize energy and nutrients efficiently for growth is inhibited to the point that additional lipid can exert only a very limited positive effect. Besides, this would also suggest that at lower temperatures, more of dietary protein was being utilized as an energy source.

The method of estimating ME, ZE + UE, and HE and nutrient and energy retention efficiencies using this comparative carcass analysis is practical for evaluation of fish diets and the results are in good agreement with those by indirect calorimetry.

Fate of Metabolizable Energy

Metabolic Rates

Heat is liberated by animals as a consequence of the metabolic transformation of dietary substrates into tissue components, as a result of tissue turnover, and as a result of physical activity. The rate at which heat is liberated is termed the metabolic rate and this varies with the qualitative and quantitative intakes of energy and nutrients and the activity of the animal. An important concept is that of basal metabolic rate which, as the term implies, is the minimum rate of metabolic activity needed to sustain the structure and function of the body tissues. The ingestion of feed increases the metabolic rate as a consequence of the extra work due to the ingestion, digestion and utilization of the diet. This increase is termed the 'heat increment of feeding' (HiE). Physical activity also increases metabolic rate due to work done against internal and external frictional forces. These three components of animal metabolism lead to the release of energy as heat from the ME derived from the diet, and clearly, energy released as heat is not available for growth (increase in body energy). Growth can occur only if the ME intake exceeds the rate of heat production. As might be anticipated, if the ME intake is less than the rate of heat production, the difference will be provided by catabolism of body tissues and weight loss will ensue. The ME minus the sum of the heat losses yields the recovered energy (RE) in animal growth.

Maintenance Energy (HEm = HEf = HeE + HjE + HcE)

Fish require a continuous supply of energy for those functions of the body immediately necessary for maintaining life (HEm) regardless of whether or not feed is being consumed. A fish deprived of feed obtains this energy (fasting heat production, HEf) by catabolizing body reserves of lipid and protein; however, in fed fish, this requirement for maintenance energy is supplied by the feed thus obviating the catabolism of body tissue. Among requirements for maintenance a major portion of the energy is spent for basal metabolism (HeE), a smaller portion of energy is also spent for voluntary or resting activity (HjE) such as minor bodily movements and muscular activity, and thermoregulation of body temperature (HcE) in the case of homeotherms.

It is difficult to ensure that the fish is in a state of muscular repose because they need to maintain their orientation in the water and this entails some muscular activity. Thus basal metabolism can be measured by extrapolation to zero activity from fish swimming at different rates. However, fish such as rainbow trout will spend considerable periods resting on the bottom of their tanks, maintaining their position in quiet water with minimal activity. The energy expenditure of fasting fish (HEf) under these conditions can be regarded as a close approximation to maintenance energy (HEm) or resting metabolism.

By definition, the basal metabolism is the minimum rate of energy expenditure needed to keep the animal alive and this has highest priority in the requirement. The basal metabolic rate is measured when the animal is in the post-absorptive state, and is in a state of muscular repose at an environmental temperature which is thermoneutral. Definition of basal metabolic rate for fish precludes the latter condition but makes it necessary to specify the temperature at which the metabolic rate was measured.

Variations in water temperature have a great effect on the fasting heat production of fish. Smith et al [1978a, b] found that increasing the temperature from 3 to 18 °C almost doubled the fasting heat production of Atlantic salmon *(Salmo salar)* and trouts. In their studies with lake trout *(Salvelinus fontinalis)* and brook trout *(Salmo trutta)* the lowest water temperature used was 6 °C and the fasting heat production of these fish was doubled by increasing the water temperature to 18 °C. Brett [1972] showed that the maintenance energy requirements of poikilothermic animals were 10–30 times lower than those of mammals which maintain body temperatures of 35 °C. However, the contribution of protein to this maintenance energy requirement seems to be higher in fish than in other animals [Luquet and Kaushik, 1979].

Heat Increment of Feeding (HiE = HdE + HrE + HwE)

Ingestion of feed by an animal which has been fasting results in an increase in the animal's heat production. This expenditure of energy due to feeding is referred to by several terms: heat increment of feeding (HiE), specific dynamic action (SDA), calorigenic effect, and dietary thermogenesis. The factors contributing to heat increment of feeding are designated as: (1) the digestion and absorption processes (HdE); (2) transformation and interconversion of the substrates and their retention in tissues (HrE), and (3) formation and excretion of metabolic wastes (HwE). The main biochemical basis for heat increment is the energy required for the ingested amino nitrogen to be deaminated and excreted (HwE) [Kleiber, 1975]. The energy expenditures associated with diet ingestion and digestion (HdE) are very small compared to that associated with metabolic work (HrE + HwE) [Brody, 1945]. The physiological basis of this increased heat production are the post-absorptive processes related to ingested diet, particularly protein-rich diet. These processes are primarily the metabolic work required for the synthesis of proteins and lipids in the tissues from the newly absorbed, feed-derived substrates such as amino acids, fatty acids and glucose and the formation of excretory nitrogen products.

Since its introduction by Rubner [1902], the term 'specific dynamic action' of diet has caused confusion, but his idea was useful because it showed that the 'chemical work of the glands' was the source of heat in contrast with the original belief that the increased heat production was due to the 'mechanical work'. This was demonstrated by feeding bone meal to dogs which did not increase heat production. This conclusion was reinforced by the observation that intravenous infusion of amino acids increased heat production to the same extent as oral administration of the amino acids [Benedict and Emmes, 1912; Borsook, 1936].

The length of time for which consumption of diet exerts an influence upon heat production depends upon many factors; chief amongst these are the quantity and quality of the diet, and the water temperature. Saunders [1963] found that oxygen consumption of Atlantic cod *(Gadus morhua)* remained above the fasting level for 7 days at 10 °C following consumption of a large meal of herring, whereas in water at 15 °C the effect lasted for only 4–5 days. Kaushik and Dabrowski [1983] similarly found that in developing larvae and juveniles, the rise in oxygen uptake corresponded more or less to the rate of transit of feedstuffs in the digestive tract. The heat increment of feeding depends to a large extent upon the balance of dietary nutrients and the plane of nutrition [Brody, 1945]. Therefore, attempts to measure the heat increment of individual feed ingredients which give a nutritionally unbalanced diet [Smith et al., 1978b; Tandler and Beamish, 1979] or measurements of effect of fish size [Beamish, 1974] and fish density [Medland and Beamish, 1985] made under forced activity conditions have very doubtful meaning.

In fish, there have been some studies on heat increment of feeding designed to separate the biochemical aspects of the post-absorptive processes from the physical or mechanical aspects of feeding and digestion. These studies involved either 'sham feeding' or feeding nondigestible materials such as kaolin or cellulose. A practical diet for largemouth bass *(Micropterus salmoides)* was diluted to 1:5 with cellulose and the effects of increasing meal volumes of the practical and diluted diets upon heat increment of feeding were compared. The difference between heat productions resulting from the two types of diet was referred to as 'mechanical SDA' [Tandler and Beamish, 1979]. The 'mechanical SDA' approached 10–30% of the total heat increment. However, Smith et al. [1978a, b] with rainbow trout, and Jobling and Davies [1980] with plaice *(Pleuronectes plattesa),* found that neither sham-feeding nor kaolin feeding increased the resting metabolic rate of their fish. Clearly, one effect of providing feed to fasting fish is an increase in physical activity, but the magnitude of this effect in relation to the physiological effects of 'normal' feed ingestion depends upon the experimental procedures employed. Sham feeding and nondigestible materials elicit minimal response compared to the use of the 'diluted' low protein diet used by Tandler and Beamish.

In mammals and birds, the heat increment of feeding is greater for high protein diets than for diets with low protein levels because of the deamination of the amino acids to be used as a source of energy and the need to detoxify the ammonia by synthesis of urea or uric acid; the energy cost of synthesis for these products being 13 and 10 kJ/g N, respectively [Martin and Blaxter, 1965]. Urea and uric acid are concentrated for excretion by the kidneys in terrestrial animals, requiring the expenditure of further energy. In contrast, as ammonia is the primary waste product of protein catabolism in fish and thus they do not require energy to detoxify or concentrate this waste [Cowey, 1975]. As a result, values for heat increment of feeding for fish are lower, ranging from 8 to 12% of IE for rainbow trout at 15 °C [Cho et al., 1982], than those encountered for terrestrial animals which can dissipate as much as 30% of the dietary energy as heat increment [Farrell, 1974]. LeGrow and Beamish [1985], however, reported that the HiE for forced-swimming rainbow trout ranged from 11.1 to 19.2% of IE. This range of values is close to that of terrestrial animals. A number of factors may have combined to elevate metabolic rate in this investigation, e.g. single fish forced to swim in a confined, electro-fenced space, and high levels of gelatin supplement to increase the dietary protein levels.

Many of the estimates of the heat increment of feeding to date are widely variable and have also created confusion and misunderstanding. The approaches used and inappropriate applications preclude generalizations concerning the loss of energy associated with this aspect of food utilization. The situation was summarized by Brett and Groves [1979]: 'It is safe to say, however, that unless serious attention to the effect of diet composition on heat increment is the aim, it is doubtful if the necessary effort to correctly partition feeding metabolism into its respective components is warranted.'

Measurement of Heat Production in Fish

Even as early as in 1914, Ege and Krogh applied the principles of bioenergetics to fishes, and later Ivlev [1939] extended these studies to carp. More recently there have been reports on energy utilization and expenditure in several species of fish [Spoor, 1946; Brett, 1962; Warren and Davies, 1967]. These early studies are primarily concerned with the energy cost of swimming by the fish and have largely ignored the level of feeding and the type of diet.

Animal calorimetry is the preferred method for nutritionists to measure energy balance of animals over the short time period for which an individual meal exerts its effect. Classically, calorimetry is the measure of heat flow between two objects and in the case of nutritional energetics, from the animal to the environment.

A direct fish calorimeter was designed by Smith et al. [1978a, b] to measure the heat production of fish. Such direct measurements of heat production deal with small temperature changes of the water as a result of changes in metabolic rates.

The indirect calorimetric method of estimating heat production depends upon the stoichiometry of nutrient catabolism and oxygen consumption: the consumption of 1 g of oxygen being associated with release of 13.6 kJ energy [Elliott and Davison, 1975]. Several indirect calorimeters (respirometers) for fish have been described [Blazka et al., 1960; Brett, 1964; Brett et al., 1971; O'Hara, 1971; Solomon and Brafield, 1972; Pierce and Wissing, 1974; Cho et al., 1975 (fig. 4), 1982; Dabrowski et al., 1986]. These calorimeters allow the oxygen consumption to be measured for fish under varying degrees of physical and/or nutritional constraints. However, complete description of the energy balance of the fish requires also accurate measurement of feed intake, fecal and other excretory losses and heat production to allow partitioning of energy on the basis of DE or ME intakes.

Measurements of energy balance using a respirometer enable nutritional evaluations of diets with different formulations. Different diets with similar levels of DE and nutrients support different levels of performance, and a frequent explanation of such differences is in the rates of heat production from the diets.

Effect of Dietary Protein on Heat Increment of Feeding

The partition of losses from dietary energy intake and the effects of dietary protein/energy balance on energy expenditure in fish are ill-defined, Fish have a lower maintenance energy requirement than higher animals because of their poikilothermic nature and body protein contributes to a great extent to these maintenance needs [Luquet and Kaushik, 1979]. In most carnivorous fish, the higher intake of protein may result in a higher expenditure of energy, because of the heat loss due to the utilization of dietary protein as an energy source.

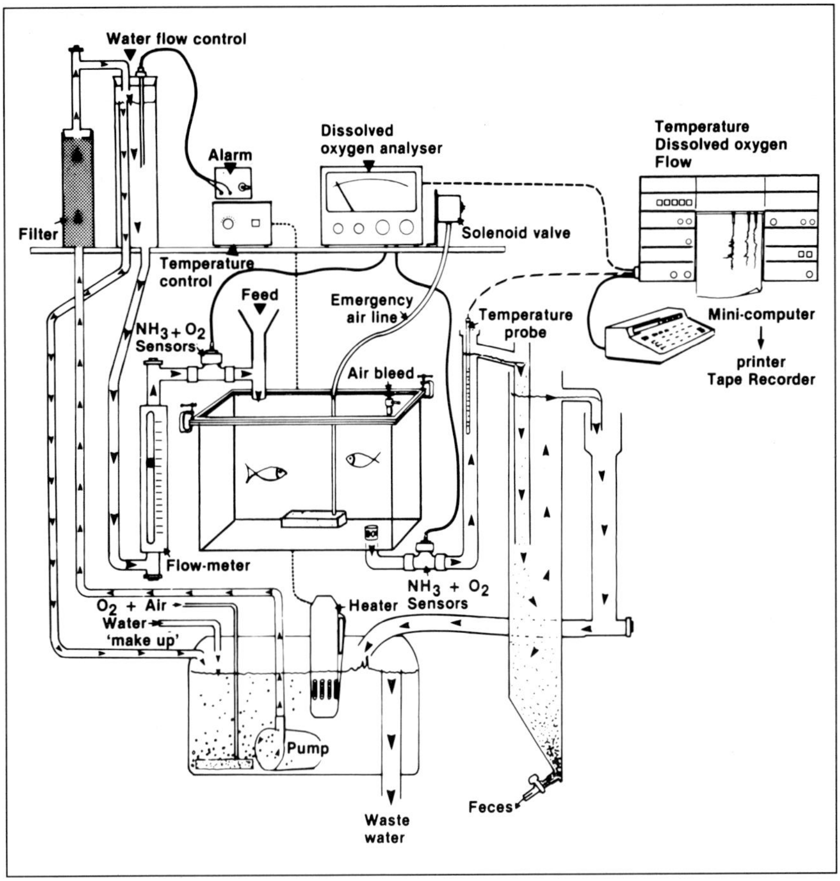

Fig. 4. Computer-controlled fish respirometer equipped with a sealed fish tank, feces settling column and instrument to measure oxygen consumption, ammonia excretion and water temperature.

In a study with rainbow trout fed three different diets of varying protein to lipid ratios, it was found that in fish fed a high protein diet, the oxygen consumption was higher than with low protein diets (table 7). These observations suggest that the energy cost of using the high protein diet exceeded that for the low protein diets. The measurements of heat increment of feeding (HiE) and fasting heat production (HEf) of the fish allow calculation of the net and recovered energy values. The highest HiE

Table 7. Influence of dietary protein and lipid levels on oxygen uptake, heat increment of feeding and the partition of DE intake by rainbow trout, showing the importance of nitrogen intake as a factor determining the heat increment of feeding[1]

Dietary protein, %	40	60	40
Dietary lipid, %	15	15	25
Oxygen uptake, g oxygen/kg BW/day			
Feeding period (mean of 8 days)	6.9	7.1	6.8
Fasting period (minimum in 3 days)	4.4	4.2	4.4
Heat increment of feeding	2.5	2.9	2.4
Energy partitioning			
Recovered energy, % of DE intake[2]	63	59	73
Heat increment of feeding			
% of DE intake[3]	11	13	8
kJ/g dig. N intake[4]	30	30	27
Fasting heat production kJ/MBW/day[5]	40	41	41

[1] Water temperature: 15 °C.
[2] Recovered energy/digestible energy intake.
[3] Heat increment/digestible energy intake.
[4] kJ heat increment/g digestible N intake.
[5] Metabolic BW (MBW) = kg $BW^{0.824}$.

loss was 13% of DE (12% of IE) with the 60% protein diet and the lowest HiE loss (8% of DE) with the high lipid diet which gave therefore the highest recovered energy value 73% of DE as a result of the direct deposition of the dietary lipid into the body without much metabolic transformations. When considered in terms of nitrogen intake, the HiE amounts to about 30 kJ/g digestible nitrogen intake at 15 °C water temperature.

Effect of Water Temperature on Heat Production

Increasing water temperature results in increased DE intake accompanied by higher total oxygen consumption for fasting heat production and heat increment of feeding (table 8). But the difference of the fasting heat production per kilogram metabolic body weight (MBW = kg $BW^{0.824}$) between 15 and 20 °C is marginal and this may indicate that the water temperature of 20 °C is above the optimum for rainbow trout which may lead to other lethal consequences rather than to an acceleration of their metabolic rates.

Table 8. Influence of water temperature on fasting heat production and on the heat increment of feeding in rainbow trout

	Water temperature, °C			
	7.5	10	15	20
Oxygen uptake, g oxygen/kg BW/day				
Feeding period (mean of 8 days)	2.2	3.9	6.3	7.1
Fasting period (minimum in 3 days)	1.3	2.7	4.5	4.1
Heat increment of feeding	0.9	1.2	1.8	3.0
Energy partitioning				
Fasting heat production, kJ/kg MBW/day	12	26	36	42
Heat increment of feeding, % of DE intake	18	12	10	13

Heat increment of feeding per unit of intake was highest at 7.5 °C (18% of DE) and lowest at 15 °C (10% of DE) which also suggests that of the temperatures used, 15 °C was closest to the optimum for efficiency of feed utilization.

Retention of Net Energy

ME taken in as diet which is not dissipated as heat is retained within the body as new tissue elements. In growing animals, the RE is partitioned between protein and lipid with the proportion of lipid increasing as the animal approaches its mature size. The relative importance of protein and lipid deposition depends upon a great number of factors in addition to the maturity of the animal. The balance of the available amino acids, particularly essential amino acids, in the dietary protein, the amount by which the dietary energy intake exceeds the maintenance requirement and the protein:energy ratio in the diet are the major factors. Proteins of high biological value may promote greater protein deposition than those of lower value. Large excesses of energy intake and improper balance of protein to energy result in the deposition of a larger proportion of the recovered energy as lipid. As the energy intake decreases, the total amount of lipid deposited decreases until, with the fish consuming less dietary energy than it expends as heat, there will be a net mobilization of lipid to support protein deposition.

Energy and Protein Retention for Growth

In almost all cases, the retention of energy as new tissue results in an increase in the weight of the animal. Weight gain of young fish is usually a reliable indicator of the adequacy of the nutritional and management regimes. Unfortunately, the rate of weight gain is not a quantitative measure of energy retention because deposition of lipid reduces the water content of the body thus changing the energy value per unit weight of the living animal. The great difference in the energy value of lipid and protein also exaggerates the difference in the energy content of body weight gain. Lipid is usually deposited in adipose tissue in association with relatively little water resulting in a heat of combustion for fish adipose tissue of 31 kJ/g, whereas protein is usually deposited in such tissues as muscle and viscera in association with a great deal of water resulting in a heat of combustion for fresh muscle tissue of 6 kJ/g.

This problem of interpreting productivity data is further complicated by the different metabolic processes by which dietary energy is stored as

Table 9. Conversion of feed and dry matter, protein and lipid of feed by rainbow trout at 15 °C for 24 weeks

	Water temp. °C	Intake/gain ratio of digestible lipid			SEM	HSD
		13%	18%	23%		
Feed	7.5	1.43	1.28	1.38	0.002	0.16
	12.5	1.14	1.02	0.95		
	17.5	1.32	1.12	1.14		
Dry matter	7.5	5.11	4.42	4.70	0.035	0.74
	12.5	3.85	3.25	2.92		
	17.5	3.92	3.35	3.22		
Protein	7.5	3.43	3.17	3.35	0.028	0.66
	12.5	2.56	2.40	2.23		
	17.5	2.82	2.68	2.56		
Lipid	7.5	1.82	1.90	2.37	0.020	0.55
	12.5	1.27	1.44	1.43		
	17.5	1.14	1.38	1.50		

108 fish × 2 rep × 24 weeks per treatment. Initial body weight: 0.078 kg/100 fish (2.32 % CV). SEM = Pooled standard error of means (df = 9); HSD = Tukey's honestly significant difference ($p < 0.05$).

either lipid or protein: the relatively simple synthesis of lipid being 74% efficient whereas the much more complex synthesis of protein being only 44% efficient as shown by Pullar and Webster [1977] for rats, and 29–45% (protein intake/gain ratio = 2.23–3.43) by Cho and Watanabe [1986] for rainbow trout (table 9). Precise measurements of the energy cost of protein synthesis, turnover or degradation in fish are however lacking [Fauconneau, 1985].

Mobilization of Body Reserve

Energy expended in swimming reduces the amount which can be retained as new body tissues. The energy expended in swimming can exceed the dietary energy intake; the balance being supplied by the mobilization of body tissue reserves. Over a long term, the energy reserves accumulated may be depleted when fish such as salmonids migrate, often without feeding, to the spawning ground.

Reproduction involves the synthesis and temporary storage of new tissues which are formed almost regardless of the level of dietary energy intake, the necessary energy being withdrawn from other body tissues if the dietary supply is insufficient. Consequently the redistribution of tissue energy which takes place in the breeding season can complicate measurements of energy balance.

Effect of Water Temperature on Energy Retention

Rainbow trout are poikilotherms and therefore water temperature is the major factor regulating their metabolic rate. The standard environmental temperature (SET) of 15 °C was recommended for rainbow trout by NRC-NAS [1973], and this temperature seems to be close to the optimum for growth, feed utilization and other considerations.

At low temperatures, basal metabolic rate of trout is reduced and they consume less feed. Therefore, the rate of gain is reduced in proportion to the reduction in temperature. At higher temperatures, rainbow trout increase their feed intake and growth. The water temperature influences the proportions of the dietary recovered energy and dissipated as heat. Increasing the water temperature from 7.5 to 20 °C increases energy retention from 37 to 51% of IE (table 10). However, Brett and Glass [1973] indicated that the active metabolic rate (swimming heat production) per unit body weight of sockeye salmon was almost unaffected by fish size in the temperature range of 5–20 °C. Since, at any given temperature, the

Table 10. Effect of temperature on partition of dietary energy in rainbow trout (% of IE)

	Water temperature, °C			
	7.5	10	15	20
Energy				
Intake (IE)	100	100	100	100
Digestible (DE)	78	78	80	80
Metabolizable (ME)	73	73	76	77
Net (NE)	58	63	67	66
Recovered (RE)	37	41	46	51
Excreted				
Fecal (FE)	22	22	20	20
Nonfecal (ZE + UE)	5	5	4	3
Heat lost				
Heat increment (HiE)	15	10	9	11
Fasting (HEf)	21	22	21	15

maintenance requirement is a fixed cost for the fish, the rate of energy retention, and hence of growth, depends mainly on the level of dietary energy intake.

Optimization of Protein and Energy Balance for Retention Efficiencies

It was noted earlier that the composition of the diet also influences energy retention: increasing dietary lipid levels from 13 to 25% of the diet results in an increase of energy retention (tables 6, 7). With a low protein diet (36% digestible protein), when the lipid levels increase from 6 to 16%, the recovered energy (RE) increased from 39% of IE to 52%. With a high-protein (47%) diet on the other hand, the increase was only from 49 to 57% of IE (table 11). Analysis of table 6 also shows that the mean ME in the diets with 3 levels of lipid were 14.4, 16.0 and 16.8 MJ/kg respectively. Increased dietary lipid levels produced increased RE as well as better protein conversion and energy retention efficiency (ERE) indicating improved utilization of protein and energy.

These results confirm the protein-sparing effect of lipids, with the most efficient combination being a diet containing 36% digestible protein and 16% lipid. Watanabe et al. [1979] found maximum protein retention

Table 11. Energy utilization by rainbow trout fed on different dietary levels of protein and lipid at 15 °C

Digestible protein, %	36			47		
Digestible lipid, %	6	11	16	6	11	16
Energy						
Intake, %	100	100	100	100	100	100
Digestible, %	73	74	80	83	84	88
Metabolizable, %	67	68	74	77	78	82
Net, %	57	60	69	64	63	70
Recovered, %	39	46	52	49	52	57
Heat lost						
Heat increment, %	10	8	5	13	15	12
Fasting, %	18	14	17	15	11	14

at an optimum protein to lipid ratio of 35% protein to 15–20% lipid. In terms of protein:energy ratios, the optimal level for maximum efficiency appears to be around 22–23 g digestible protein/MJ DE [Cho and Woodward, 1989]. With the use of digestible carbohydrates like gelatinized starch, similar effects on protein and energy retention efficiencies were found by Kaushik and Oliva-Teles [1985].

Comparison of Efficiencies of Protein and Energy Retention between Fish and Poultry

A schematic partitioning of protein and energy flow in rainbow trout is presented in figure 5. Fishes are generally considered more efficient feed converters than other farm animals in spite of the fact that cultivable carnivorous fish consume diets with much higher protein and energy densities. By means of a comparison of the protein and energy utilization, a critical evaluation is presented herein of the diet utilization by the salmonids and poultry.

In table 12 is presented a comparison of the efficiencies of protein and energy retention between rainbow trout [Cho et al., 1982] and broiler chickens [Leeson and Summers, 1980]. When fed a high-protein, low-lipid diet (diet B), rainbow trout retain a smaller proportion of ingested protein than chickens. This is because almost three quarters of the total energy loss by rainbow trout fed high protein diets is derived from dietary protein. By

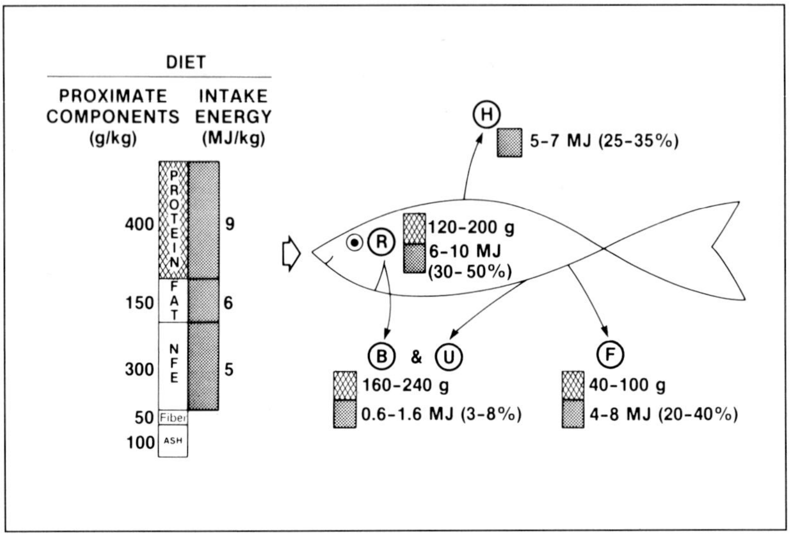

Fig. 5. Schematic budgeting of protein and energy flow in fish. F = Fecal loss; B and U = branchial and urinary losses; H = heat loss; R = retention in body. The vertical bars on the left depict proximate and energy components of a fish diet. All values shown are absolute values and numbers in parentheses are percentages of total energy intake.

contrast, only about 40% of the total energy lost as heat by the broiler chicken is derived from dietary protein. The situation for the rainbow trout is improved if the diet contains a higher proportion of the nonprotein energy as lipid (diet A); in these trout, a greater proportion of the total energy loss is derived from nonprotein energy constituents of the diet than is the case for trout fed the 'high-protein' diet. The practice of formulating high protein salmonid diets, therefore, does not promote optimal retention of dietary protein or of total energy by the fish.

Energy and Protein Requirements of Fish with Particular Reference to Rainbow Trout (Salmo gairdneri)

Quantitative estimates of dietary energy requirements which are applicable to production conditions are scarce at present and, furthermore, the information which is available is mostly for salmonids, particularly

Table 12. Estimation of dietary nitrogen and energy utilization by broiler chicken and rainbow trout[1]

		Nitrogen g	Energy		
			total diet MJ	protein MJ	nonprotein MJ
Broiler chicken diet (20% crude protein/6% fat)[2]					
Intake, gross		225	94	33	61
Retained, carcass	% of intake	37	43	–	–
	% of retained			30	70
Excretion and heat	% of intake	63	57	–	–
	% of losses			39	61
Trout diet A (34% dig. protein/22% dig. fat)					
Intake, gross		6.2	2.2	0.9	1.3
Retained, carcass	% of intake	47	50	–	–
	% of retained			39	61
Excretion and heat	% of intake	53	50	–	–
	% of losses			45	55
Trout diet B (55% dig. protein/13% dig. fat)					
Intake, gross		10.0	2.4	1.5	0.9
Retained, carcass	% of intake	34	43	–	–
	% of retained			49	51
Excretion and heat	% of intake	66	57	–	–
	% of losses			74	26

[1] Body weight: 50–3,500 g/bird in 70 days; 1–100 g/fish in 140 days. Trout data obtained at 15 °C water temperature.
[2] Leeson and Summers [1980].

rainbow trout. The influence of age, exercise and of environmental factors on the energy requirements has been studied in laboratory settings, but the significance of these energy expectations under aquaculture conditions are not clearly defined.

The important part of energy requirement is the amount of energy needed for maintaining life processes, since body tissues are catabolized to meet this energy requirement if the dietary intake of 'energy-yielding' nutrients is not sufficient. In a practical sense, the minimum dietary energy requirement is to satisfy the animal's energy needs for maintenance

(HEm). Unlike other nutrients, we can hardly talk of a minimum recommended energy requirement for fish production (RE) as such, because any net excess dietary energy over the heat lost under maintenance conditions may potentially be stored as protein and lipid in the body. However, this excess chemical energy must be provided in an appropriate balance among protein, lipid and carbohydrate in the diet to maximize the efficiency of growth and reproduction.

The fasting heat production due to energy expenditure for basal metabolism and voluntary activity can account for about 70% of total heat production (HE) under feeding regimes. The heat increment of feeding for a maintenance ration is approximately one third of the total heat increment (HiE) and the rest (two thirds) is the heat expended in the anabolism of the productive gain.

An understanding of this general framework of fish energetics allows the construction of a quantitative model, as shown in table 13, for 10 fish growing from 1 to 101 g. The production of 1 kg biomass gain (100 g/fish)

Table 13. An example of estimating energy requirement to produce 1 kg biomass of rainbow trout[1]

	Recovered	Losses		Note
		heat	excretion	
Carcass energy 100 g ×10 fish	8.0			1 kg biomass with 70% moisture
Fasting oxygen		4.4		2.73 g oxygen or 37 kJ ($kgBW^{0.824}$) per day
Heat increment digestible of feeding		1.7		30 kJ/g nitrogen intake
Nonfecal losses			0.8	25 kJ/g nonfecal nitrogen losses
Fecal loss			5.0	ADC (energy) = 0.75 by rainbow trout
Total	8.0 19.9 MJ/kg feed	6.1	5.8	DP/DE = 23 g/MJ feed/gain = 1.0

[1] Growth period: 1–101 g fish in 140 days. Water temperature: 15 °C under laboratory conditions. RE = 8.0, NE = 12.4, ME = 14.1, DE = 14.9, and IE = 19.9 MJ, respectively. ADC (energy) = Apparent digestibility coefficient of energy.

requires 4.4 MJ of heat energy for maintenance (HEm), and 1.7 MJ of heat energy (HiE) as the cost of utilizing dietary nutrients (mainly protein) for both life-maintaining process and growth. One kg of rainbow trout biomass contains approximately 300 g dry matter (165 g protein, 105 g lipid and 30 g ash) which is equivalent to 8 MJ of chemical energy. Thus, 14.1 MJ of ME are required for the production of 1 kg of trout biomass. With a feed conversion of 1.0 (feed:gain) the gross energy intake would be 19.9 MJ (or 14.9 MJ DE), the excretory losses would be 0.8 MJ of branchial (ZE) plus urinary (UE) and 5 MJ fecal (FE) energy losses.

Although the above example is valid only for the conditions specified, some of the components of this energy model can be varied. For example, the energy losses due to the heat increment of feeding and nonfecal loss are dependent on the level and balance of protein and energy in the diet. Salmonid production diets including 'starter feed' should not provide more than 25 g digestible protein (DP) per MJ of digestible energy (DE) intake (e.g. 373 g DP; 14.9 MJ/kg), however, finishing 'grower' diets should not provide less than 20 g DP/MJ DE intake (e.g. 298 g DP; 14.9 MJ/kg). Excess protein intake in relation to energy intake increases the nonfecal loss, and the heat increment of feeding.

By contrast, the requirement of total energy to produce 1 kg of fish is relatively independent of water temperature, since as temperature increases, energy intake is increased and, consequently, the growth rate increases. Furthermore, different species of fish with similar carcass composition and metabolic rate may have similar energy requirements under intensive culture conditions.

The recommended levels of energy and protein:energy ratios for salmonid diets are shown in table 14. These levels have been employed for salmonid diets in Ontario, Canada, for many years (table 15). For clarity of

Table 14. Recommended levels of energy and protein for salmonid diets

Gross intake energy	17–20 MJ/kg feed
Digestible energy[1]	14–17 MJ/kg feed
Metabolizable energy	13–16 MJ/kg feed
Digestible protein per MJ digestible energy	22–25 g/MJ

[1] Include 4–7 MJ energy of lipid origin (fish oil) per kg feed. The levels of energy and protein may be adjusted according to water temperature and projected growth rate.

diet formulation, the recommended levels are based on MJ, kg and g rather than in terms of percentage of the feed. However, it is essential that the requirements for biologically utilizable energy and the nutrient intakes, not the weight of feed, must be the main considerations by fish culturists, when determining the daily feed allowance.

Table 15. Purified and practical reference test diets for salmonids[1]

Ingredient	Purified (C102) g/kg diet	Practical (C202) g/kg diet
Casein, vitamin-free or high N	400	–
Gelatin	40	–
Starch, raw	115	–
Dextrin, white	90	–
D-Glucose	50	–
Cellulose	30	–
L-Arginine · HCl	10	–
DL-Methionine	5	–
Fish meal, herring, 70% CP	–	300
Soybean meal, 48% CP	–	170
Corn gluten meal, 60% CP	–	130
Wheat middlings, 17% CP	–	250
Vitamin and mineral premixes	110[2]	30[3]
Fish oil, herring[4]	150	120

[1] All diets can be steam-pelleted at 0.4–0.7 kg/cm^2 without addition of water.

[2] Milligrams/kilogram diet except as noted: retinyl acetate 7,000 IU; cholecalciferol 3,000 IU; *all-rac*-alpha-tocopheryl acetate 200 IU; menadione sodium bisulfite 50; thiamine·HCl 40; riboflavin 60; *D*-Ca-pantothenate 200; biotin 0.5; folic acid 20; cyanocobalamin 0.2; niacin 300; pyridoxine·HCl 40; myoinositol 500; ascorbic acid 500; choline dihydrogen citrate 11,000; dibasic calcium phosphate (23% Ca, 18% P) 30,000; calcium carbonate (40% Ca) 3,000; NaCl 15,000; potassium sulfate (45% K) 20,000; magnesium sulfate (20% Mg) 10,000; ferrous sulfate (21% Fe) 700; manganous sulfate (33% Mn) 300; zinc sulfate (36% Zn) 550; cupric sulfate (25% Cu) 160; cobalt chloride (25% Co) 26; potassium iodide (76% I) 15; sodium selenite (42% Se) 2.5; cellulose.

[3] Milligrams/kilogram diet except as noted: vitamin A (as acetate) 4,000 IU; vitamin D_3 2,500 IU; vitamin E (as *dl*-alpha-tocopheryl acetate) 90 IU; vitamin K (as menadione sodium bisulfate) 20; vitamin B_{12} 0.03; ascorbic acid 400; biotin 0.2; folic acid 10; niacin 200; *D*-Ca-pantothenate 70; pyridoxine·HCl 15; riboflavin 20; thiamin·HCl 20; choline chloride 1,000; $CuSO_4 \cdot 5H_2O$ 25; $FeSO_4 \cdot 7H_2O$ 63; $MnSO_4 \cdot H_2O$ 86; KI 8; $ZnSO_4 \cdot H_2O$ 144; NaCl 3,000; wheat middlings.

[4] Deaerated with nitrogen and stabilized with 0.05% ethoxyquin.

Protein: Energy Balance in Formulation and Evaluation of Fish Diets

The final objectives of investigating the nutritional energetics are in applications for diet formulation and evaluation, estimation of growth and protein retention, and relative comparison of the productivity of fishes with other agricultural animals. The essential thrust of such studies is to provide bases of procedures for the formulation and evaluation of production diets on the concept that there is an optimum balance of energy and nutrients to promote maximum utilization of dietary protein and energy. On the basis of the foregoing observations, the following practical applications can be made.

Importance of DE in Feed Formulation

The value of a diet depends upon the levels and availabilities of the more than 40 nutrients which have been shown necessary for fishes. But the energy value of the diet is most important because this determines the amount of diet consumed by the fish since they adjust their feed intake to satisfy their needs for energy. In most cases as the digestible energy levels increase, the voluntary feed intakes of fish decrease. Fish like other animals eat to satisfy their energy requirements [Cowey, 1975; Kaushik et al., 1981]. Thus the actual intake of all the other nutrients is regulated by the available energy level of the diet. Hence measurement of digestibility gives a good indication of the nutritional quality of feed ingredients, allowing a rational basis for the formulation of diets to meet specified standards of available nutrient levels.

However, this simple measure does not provide any indication of the interactions which can influence the proportion of the dietary energy intake which is retained by the fish and used for growth. It might be worth investigating the biologically utilizable energy (ME or NE) content of a diet to predict its productivity.

The metabolic losses which occur after digestion of the diet, depend upon the appropriateness of the balance between protein and energy, the amount of feeding, and upon the physiological status of the fish. None of these factors can be directly attributed to the inherent characteristics of the feed ingredients included in the diet, but depend upon the skill of the nutritionist in formulating the feed ingredients into a diet balanced with respect to the animal's nutrient needs.

Practical Approach to Feed Evaluation

Although ME values are frequently used to compare the quality of feed ingredients in diets for other species of livestock such as poultry, the practical difficulties of measuring the nonfecal losses by fish suggest that both feed ingredients and compound diets should be compared for fish using DE values. Among the losses from the feed intake, the fecal loss (20–40%) is the primary reason for variation in the nutritional values of diets.

Table 16 shows a simplified approach to feed evaluation [Cho and Kaushik, 1985; Cho, 1987]. For practical applications such as feed formulation and evaluation and estimation and partition of dietary energy for a species of fish can be obtained in a more simpler way than as described in the previous sections. These procedures can be carried out by sampling diet, feces and carcass and analyzing the proximate composition and gross energy. The advantage of using DE values to compare different feed ingredients is that these values are additive: if the formula of the diet and DE values of the ingredients are known, the DE value of the mixed diet can be calculated. Only if the diets formulated on the basis of digestibility fail to support standard levels of productivity the complex issue of post-absorptive losses should be examined. Measurements of these post-absorptive losses require much more sophisticated facilities and employ more invasive techniques which impose more stress on the fish, than the simpler measurement of digestibility.

The effectiveness of diets formulated on the basis of the digestibilities of the energy and other nutrients in the feed ingredients can be evaluated

Table 16. Partition of dietary energy by digestibility and comparative carcass analysis

1	Measure digestible N (DN) and energy (DE) intake
2	Measure recovered N (RN) and energy (RE) gains in carcass
3	Measure carcass N (RNf) and energy (REf = HEf = HEm) losses during fasting
4	Calculate nonfecal N (UN + ZN) = DN – RN
	Nonfecal energy (UE + ZE) = 24.9 (UN + ZN)[1]
	Metabolizable energy (ME) = DE – (UE + ZE)
	Heat production (HE) = ME – RE
	Heat increment (HiE) = ME – RE – REf
	Net energy (NE) = ME – HiE

[1] 24.9 kJ/g ammonia-N including some urea-N.

by determination of weight gain, feed efficiency and body composition of fish received the diets under a particular culture regime. These parameters are the ultimate goals of fish production.

References

Beamish, F.W.H.: Apparent specific dynamic action of largemouth bass, Micropterus salmoides. J. Fish. Res. Board Can. *31:* 1763–1769 (1974).

Benedict, F.G.; Emmes, L.E.: The influence upon metabolism of non-oxidizable material in the intestinal tract. Am. J. Physiol. *30:* 197 (1912).

Blazka, P.; Volf, M.; Cephela, M.: A new type of respirometer for the determination of the metabolism of fish in an active state. Physiol. Bohemoslov *9:* 553–558 (1960).

Bligh, E.G.; Dyer, W.J.: A rapid method of total lipid extraction and purification. Can. J. Biochem. Physiol. *37:* 911–917 (1959).

Borsook, H.: The specific dynamic action of protein and amino acids in animals. Bio. Rev. *11:* 147–180 (1936).

Brafield, A.E.; Llewellyn, M.J.: Animal energetics (Blackie & Son, Glasgow 1982).

Brett, J.R.: Some considerations in the study of respiratory metabolism in fish, particularly salmon. J. Fish. Res. Board Can. *19:* 1025–1038 (1962).

Brett, J.R.: The respiratory metabolism and swimming performance of young sockey salmon. J. Fish. Res. Board Can. *21:* 1183–1226 (1964).

Brett, J.R.: The metabolic demand for oxygen in fish, particularly salmonids and a comparison with other vertebrates. Respir. Physiol. *14:* 151–170 (1972).

Brett, J.R.; Glass, N.R.: Metabolic rates and critical swimming speeds of sockeye salmon *(Oncorhynchus nerka)* in relation to size and temperature. J. Fish. Res. Board Can. *30:* 379–387 (1973).

Brett, J.R.; Groves, T.D.D.: Physiological energetics; in Fish physiology, vol.VIII, Hoar, Randall, Brett, pp. 279–352 (Academic Press, New York 1979).

Brett, J.R.; Sutherland, D.B.; Heritage, G.D.: An environmental-control tank for the synchronous study of growth and metabolism of young salmon. Fish Res. Board Can. Tech. Rep., No. 283 (1971).

Brett, J.R.; Zala, C.A.: Daily pattern of nitrogen excretion and oxygen consumption of sockeye salmon *(Oncorhynchus nerka)* under controlled condition. J. Fish. Res. Board Can. *32:* 2479–2486 (1975).

Brody, S.: Bioenergetics and growth (Reinhold, New York 1945); reprint (Hafner Press, New York 1974).

Cho, C.Y.: Studies on nutritional energetics and protein utilization in rainbow trout (*Salmo gairdneri* Richardson), p. 137 (Kyushu University, Fukuoka 1987).

Cho, C.Y.; Bayley, H.S.; Slinger, S.J.: An automated fish repirometer for nutrition studies. Proc. 28th Annu. Meet. of Can. Conf. for Fish. Res., Vancouver 1975.

Cho, C.Y.; Bayley, H.S.; Slinger, S.J.: Energy metabolism in growing rainbow trout: partition of dietary energy in high protein and high fat diets. Proc. 7th Symp. of Energy Metabolism, Vichy 1976, pp. 299–302.

Cho, C.Y.; Kaushik, S.J.: Effects of protein intake on metabolizable and net energy values of fish diets; in Cowey, Mackie, Bell, Nutrition and feeding in fish, pp. 95–117 (Academic Press, London 1985).

Cho, C.Y.; Slinger, S.J.; Bayley, H.S.: Bioenergetics of salmonid fishes: energy intake, expenditure and productivity. Compar. Biochem. Physiol. *73B:* 25–41 (1982).

Cho, C.Y.; Watanabe, T.: Dietary energy and lipid requirements of rainbow trout *(Salmo gairdneri)* at different water temperatures. Proc. 10th Int. Symp. on Energy Metabolism, Airlie 1986.

Cho, C.Y.; Woodward, B.: Studies on the protein-to-energy ratio in diets for rainbow trout *(Salmo gairdneri).* Proc. 11th Symp. on Energy Metabolism, Lunteren 1988, pp. 37–40. EAAP Publ. 43 (Pudoc, Wageningen 1989).

Choubert, G., Jr.; Noue, J. de la; Luquet, P.: Continuous quantitative automatic collector for fish feces. Prog. Fish-Cult. *41:* 64–67 (1979).

Cowey, C.B.: Aspects of protein utilization by fish. Proc. Nutr. Soc. *34:* 57–63 (1975).

Cowey, C.B.; Luquet, P.: Physiological basis of protein requirements of fishes. Critical evaluation of allowances. Proc. IV Symp. Protein Metabolism, Clermont-Ferrand, INRA 1983, pp. 365–384.

Dabrowski, K.; Kaushik, S.J.; Bergot, P.: Active metabolism in young coregonids: a new approach involving oxygen consumption and ammonia excretion. Arch. Hydrobiol. Beih. *22:* 161–169 (1986).

Diggs, B.G.; Becher, D.E.; Jensen, A.H.; Norton, H.W.: Energy value of various feeds for the young pig. J. Anim. Sci. *24:* 555–558 (1965).

Edin, H.: Orienterande forsok over anvandbarheten av en pa 'ledkroppsprincipen' grundad metod att bestamma en foder- blandings smaltbarhed. Centralanstalten for forsoksvasendet pa jordbruksomradet. Stockholm Medd. *165:* 1–28 (1918).

Ege, R.; Krogh, A.: On the relation between the temperature and the respiratory exchange in fishes. Int. Rev. ges. Hydrobiol. Hydrogr. *1:* 48–55 (1914).

Elliott, J.M.; Davison, W.: Energy equivalents of oxygen consumption in animal energetics. Oecologia *19:* 195–201 (1975).

Fange, R.; Grove, D.: Digestion; in Hoar, Randall, Brett, Fish physiology, vol. VIII, pp. 162–260 (Academic Press, New York 1979).

Farrell, D.J.: General principles and assumptions of calorimetry; in Energy requirements of poultry, pp. 1–24 (British Poultry Science, 1974).

Fauconneau, B.: Protein synthesis and protein deposition in fish; in Cowey, Mackie, Bell, Nutrition and feeding in fish, pp. 95–117 (Academic Press, London 1985).

Fauconneau, B.; Choubert, G.; Blanc, D.; Breque, J.; Luquet, P.: Influence of environmental temperature on flow rate of foodstuffs through the gastrointestinal tract of rainbow trout. Aquaculture *34:* 27–39 (1983).

Forster, R.P.; Goldstein, L.: Formation of excretory products; in Hoar, Randall, Fish physiology, vol. I, pp. 313–350 (Academic Press, New York 1969).

Hunn, J.B.: Urine flow rate of fresh water of salmonids. Prog. Fish-Cult. *44:* 119–121 (1981).

Ivlev, V.S.: Energy balance in the carp. Zoll. Zh. *18:* 303–318 (1939).

Jobling, M.; Davies, P.S.: Effects of feeding on metabolic rate, and the specific dynamic action in plaice, *Pleuronectes platessa* L. J. Fish Biol. *16:* 629–638 (1980).

Kaushik, S.J.: Influence of nutritional status on the daily patterns of nitrogen excretion in the carp (*Cyprinus carpio* L.) and the rainbow trout (*Salmo gairdneri* R.). Reprod. Nutr. Dev. *20:* 1751–1765 (1980).

Kaushik, S.J.: Influence of a rise in temperature on nitrogen excretion of rainbow trout (*Salmo gairdneri* R.); in Tiews, Aquaculture in heated effluents and recirculation systems, vol. I, pp. 77–89 (Bundesforschungsanstalt für Fischerei, Berlin 1981).
Kaushik, S.J.; Dabrowski, K.: Postprandial metabolic changes in larval and juvenile carp *(Cyprinus carpio).* Reprod. Nutr. Dev. *23:* 223–234 (1983).
Kaushik, S.J.; Dabrowski, K.; Luquet, P.: Patterns of nitrogen excretion and oxygen consumption during ontogenesis of common carp *(Cyprinus carpio).* Can. J. Fish. Aquat. Sci. *39:* 1095–1105 (1982).
Kaushik, S.J.; Luquet, P.; Blanc, D.: Usefulness of feeding protein and non-protein calories apart in studies on energy-protein interrelationships in rainbow trout. Ann. Zootech. *30:* 3–11 (1981).
Kaushik, S.J.; Oliva-Teles, A.: Effect of digestible energy on nitrogen and energy balance in rainbow trout. Aquaculture *50:* 89–101 (1985).
Kleiber, M.: The fire of life (Kleiber, New York 1975).
Krebs, H.A.; Kornberg, H.L.: Energy transformations in living matter (Springer, Berlin 1957).
Leeson, S.; Summers, J.D.: Production and carcass characteristics of the broiler chicken. Poultry Sci. *59:* 786–798 (1980).
LeGrow, S.M.; Beamish, F.W.H.: Influence of dietary protein and lipid on apparent heat increment of rainbow trout, *Salmo gairdneri.* Can. J. Fish. Aquat. Sci. *43:* 19–25 (1985).
Luquet, P.; Kaushik, S.J.: Besoins en proteines et en acides amines; in Nutrition des poissons. Actes du coll. (CNERNA, Paris 1979).
Martin, A.K.; Blaxter, K.L.: The energy cost of urea synthesis in sheep; in Blaxter, Energy metabolism, pp. 83–91 (Academic Press, New York 1965).
Medland, T.E.; Beamish, F.W.H.: The influence of diet and fish density on apparent heat increment in rainbow trout, *Salmo gairdneri.* Aquaculture *47:* 1–10 (1985).
Needham, J.: Chemical embryology, vol. II (Cambridge University Press, Cambridge 1931).
Nose, T.: On the digestion of food protein by gold fish (*Carassius auratus* L). and rainbow trout (*Salmo irideus* G.). Bull. Freshwater Fish. Res. Lab. *10:* 23–28 (1960).
NRC-NAS: Nutrient requirements of coldwater fishes. Nutrient requirement of domestic animals, No. 11 (National Academy Press, Washington 1973).
NRC-NAS: Nutritional energetics of domestic animals and glossary of energy terms; 2nd rev. ed. (National Academy Press, Washington 1981a).
NRC-NAS: Nutrient requirements of coldwater fishes. Nutrient requirement of domestic animals, No. 16 (National Academy Press, Washington 1981b).
Ogino, C.; Kakino, J.; Chen, M.S.: Determination of metabolic fecal nitrogen and endogenous nitrogen excretion of carp. Bull. Jap. Soc. Sci. Fish. *39:* 519–523 (1973).
O'Hara, J.: A continuously monitored respiration chamber for fish. Water Res., vol. 5, pp. 143–145 (Pergamon Press, Oxford 1971).
Pierce, R.J.; Wissing, T.E.: Energy cost of food utilization in the bluegill. Trans. Am. Fish, Soc. *103:* 38–45 (1974).
Pilgrim, R.L.C.: Waste of carbon and of energy in nitrogen excretion. Nature *173:* 491 (1954).
Pullar, J.D.; Webster, A.J.F.: The energy cost of fat and protein deposition in the rat. Br. J. Nutr. *37:* 355–363 (1977).

Rubner, M.: Die Gesetze des Energieverbrauchs bei der Ernährung (Deutsche, Leipzig 1902).
Saunders, R.L.: Respiration of the atlantic cod. J. Fish. Res. Board Can. *20:* 373–386 (1963).
Schroedinger, E.: What is life (Cambridge University Press, Cambridge 1944).
Smith, R.R.: A method for measuring digestibility and metabolizable energy of feeds. Prog. Fish-Cult. *33:* 132–134 (1971).
Smith, R.R.; Peterson, M.C.; Allred, A.C.: Effect of leaching on apparent digestion coefficients of feedstuffs for salmonids. Prog. Fish-Cult. *42:* 195–199 (1980).
Smith, R.R.; Rumsey, G.L.; Scott, M.L.: Net energy maintenance requirement of salmonids as measured by direct calorimetry: effect of body size and environmental temperature. J. Nutr. *108:* 1017–1024 (1978a).
Smith, R.R.; Rumsey, G.L.; Scott, M.L.: Heat increment associated with dietary protein, fat and carbohydrate and complete diets in salmonids: comparative energetic efficiency. J. Nutr. *108:* 1025–1032 (1978b).
Solomon, D.J.; Brafield, A.E.: The energetics of feeding metabolism and growth of perch (*Perca fluviatilis* L.). J. Anim. Ecol. *41:* 699–718 (1972).
Spoor, W.A.: A quantitative study of the relationship between activity and oxygen consumption of the goldfish and its application to the measurement of respiratory metabolism in fishes. Biol. Bull. *91:* 312–325 (1946).
Steel, R.G.D.; Torrie, J.H.: Principles and procedures of statistics, with special references to the biological sciences, pp. 109–110 (McGraw-Hill, New York 1960).
Tandler, A.; Beamish, F.W.H.: Mechanical and biochemical components of apparent specific dynamic action in largemouth bass, *Micropterus salmoides lacepe lacepede.* J. Fish Biol. *14:* 343–350 (1979).
Warren, C.E.; Davis, G.E.: Laboratory studies on the feeding, bioenergetics, and growth of fish; in Gerking, The biological basis of freshwater fish production, pp. 175–214 (Blackwell Scientific Publications, Oxford 1967).
Watanabe, T.; Takeuchi, T.; Ogino, C.: Studies on the sparing effect of lipids on dietary protein in rainbow trout *(Salmo gairdneri).* Proc. World Symp. on Finfish Nutrition and Fishfeed Technology, Hamburg 1979, vol. I, pp. 113–125.
Windell, J.T.; Foltz, J.W.; Sarokon, J.A.: Methods of fecal collection and nutrient leaching in digestibility studies. Prog. Fish-Cult. *40:* 51–55 (1978).

C.Y. Cho, Dr. Agro., Fisheries Branch, Ontario Ministry of Natural Resources
and Department of Nutritional Sciences, University of Guelph,
Guelph, Ont. N1G 2W1 (Canada)

Bourne GH (ed): Aspects of Food Production, Consumption and Energy Values.
World Rev Nutr Diet. Basel, Karger, 1990, vol 61, pp 173–208

Metabolic Adaptation to Decreases in Energy Intake Due to Changes in the Energy Cost of Low Energy Expenditure Regimen[1]

Lars Garby

Department of Physiology, University of Odense, Denmark

Contents

[1] This paper was originally prepared under author's contract with the Food Policy and Nutrition Division of the Food and Agriculture Organization of the United Nations (FAO), and is published by permission of that Organization.

1. Introduction

The concept that human beings have requirements of food energy intake is basic to a number of activities of international and national organizations involved in food production and health.

The concept of energy requirements is closely related to the concept of energy expenditure. In fact, estimations of prevalence of energy intakes below requirements (= undernutrition) are based on measurements of energy expenditure [15] under prescribed conditions.

Energy expenditure of man is related to several factors. Some of them, e.g. physical activity, body mass and composition, ambient temperature and relation to recent food intake, are well known, and on the whole well understood, and there is good evidence to believe that they are causally related to the energy expenditure: the energy expenditure *depends* on these factors. Other factors, such as sex and age, are related to energy expenditure, but their effects may be secondary to, for example, body composition: the energy expenditure then does not *depend* on these factors.

It has been suggested – most recently in a series of papers by Sukhatme [39, 40] and by Miller [33], but some of the suggestions can be traced back to very early literature – that the energy expenditure of a subject with given physical activity, body mass and composition, ambient temperature and relation to recent food intake depends also on the previous history of food energy intake. There are several different forms of this suggestion, but if they are formulated in such a way that the dependence on the previous history of food energy intake is due to changes in the efficiency with which the body utilizes the chemical energy in the food, then the suggestions become equivalent to *an hypothesis of a physiological adaptation with no costs.* This hypothetical phenomenon has also been called metabolic adaptation, a terminology which is reasonable insofar as most of the energy transformations of importance in this context are chemical, or physicochemical, in nature.

The question of whether the phenomenon of metabolic adaptation exists or not or, rather, to what extent it may exist, is of direct relevance to present FAO methodology for estimation of prevalence of undernutrition in communities [15].

For a variety of reasons, the concept of metabolic adaptation and its relation to experimental observations is not simple. The present paper is an attempt to clarify the concept and, in particular, relate it to what can be observed experimentally. In addition, comments will be made concerning the consequences, in terms of public health, of the concept. Finally, a number of experimental observations, relevant to the concept, will be reviewed.

2. Concepts and Mechanisms of Metabolic Adaptation

The relation between a theoretical concept and the observations predicted by it is not always unique. The predicted observations may be interpreted in terms other than that of the theory. Confirmation, or rejection, of the hypothesis of metabolic adaptation therefore requires that the relation between the concept and the observations is analysed in detail.

The first part of this section deals with the concept of energy expenditure and how this can be measured. The second part deals with the relation between energy expenditure and the efficiency with which energy is transduced, or transformed, in the human body. Two concepts are described in detail, i.e. that of coupled processes and that of stationary energy potentials. A subsection is devoted to the regulation and control of the energy potentials in the body, i.e. the processes that form the basis for the concept of metabolic adaptation.

2.1. Energy Conservation: Energy Expenditure

In this subsection I define the expression *energy expenditure* and relate it to observable quantities. The First Law of Thermodynamics states that energy is conserved and this leads to the following statement for the human body:

– Rate of change of energy content + flow of energy into the body = flow of energy out of the body. (1)

Since, for practically all purposes, we can neglect the contributions of kinetic energy and potential energy to the *total energy*, the energy in equation 1 is the *internal energy*. Equation 1 can then be formulated [18] in the following six terms (see equation 2 below): (i) the rate of change of body thermal energy; (ii) the rate of change of amount of matter in the body and the energy associated with this matter; (iii) the flow of matter into the body and the energy associated with this matter; (iv) the flow of matter out of the body and the energy associated with this matter; (v) the flow of heat out of the body, and (vi) the rate of work performed by the body on its surroundings. We have

$$\underset{\text{(i)}}{-\overline{C} \times d\overline{T}/dt} \quad \underset{\text{(ii)}}{-\Sigma dN \times h/dt} \quad \underset{\text{(iii)}}{+\sum_{in} \dot{n} \times h} \quad \underset{\text{(iv)}}{-\sum_{out} \dot{n} \times h} = \underset{\text{(v)}}{\dot{q}} + \underset{\text{(vi)}}{\dot{w}} \tag{2}$$

where $\overline{C}$ is the average heat capacity of the body, $\overline{T}$ is the average body temperature, t is time, N is the amount of matter in the body with energy h (per unit of matter), $\dot{n}$ is the flow of matter with energy h, $\dot{q}$ is the flow of heat out of the body and $\dot{w}$ is the rate of work performed by the body on its surroudings.[2] The summation is over all kinds of matter, i.e. all chemical species.

Inspection of equation 2 immediately suggests a rational definition of the term energy expenditure as the sum $(\dot{q} + \dot{w} + \sum_{out} \dot{n} \cdot h)$, i.e. as *the total flow of energy out of the system.* However, as will be shown below, a slightly different definition is better suited to most practical situations.

A large number of terms in equation 2, i.e. in the terms ii–iv, are, in general, not observable. However, as will be shown below, most of them can be ignored because they are quantitatively insignificant. In order to develop equation 2, I will start with the simplest case and work out the more complicated and realistic cases subsequently. The aim is to obtain an operational definition of the term energy expenditure and to analyse the situations where this can be observed by different methodologies.

Case 1. In this case we assume (a) that only one substrate, e.g. glucose, and oxygen flows into the body and that this substrate undergoes complete oxidation (=combustion) with subsequent excretion of the products and (b) that all the intensive properties of the system (concentrations, electrical potentials, pressures and temperatures) are time independent, i.e. that the whole system is in a stationary state. The first two terms in equation 2 are therefore equal to zero and we have that:

$$\dot{n}_s \cdot h_s + \dot{n}_{O_2} \cdot h_{O_2} - \dot{n}_{CO_2} \cdot h_{CO_2} - \dot{n}_{H_2O} \cdot h_{H_2O} = \dot{q} + \dot{w}, \tag{3}$$

[2] A few comments are needed with respect to the term $\dot{w}$, i.e. the rate of performance of work by the body on its surroundings. This usually takes the form of compression of materials (ground, chair) and movements of air molecules and material bodies. It can in principle be expressed as force times length per unit of time. The term physical activity is used among physiologists to denote movements of the body itself and the relation between the two terms is not simple. In general, the term $\dot{w}$ is much smaller than the term $\dot{q}$ (see further section 3.2.2).

where s stands for substrate. According to standard chemical thermodynamics, the sum of the four terms on the left side is equal to $-\dot{n}_s \cdot \Delta h_s$, where Δh_s stands for the energy of reaction (= combustion) of the substrate, so that:

$$-\dot{n}_s \cdot \Delta h_s = \dot{q} + \dot{w}. \quad (4)$$

In this case, substrate flows into the system and cannot, by virtue of assumption *b* above, accumulate. The *energy expenditure* is given directly as the sum ($\dot{q} + \dot{w}$) by *direct calorimetry*. However, the energy expenditure in this case is also given by the term $\dot{n}_s \cdot \Delta h_s$, which can be observed by *indirect calorimetry*: the stoichiometry of the combustion reaction is known and the flow $\dot{n}_s$ can be calculated from the flow $\dot{n}_{O_2}$, a generally observable quantity. The *heat production* in the body is, by virtue of assumption *b* above, given by $\dot{q}$ and can only be calculated when $\dot{w}$ can be measured. A body at rest performs no external work and $\dot{w} = 0$.

Case 2. In this case, we retain the assumption of stationarity, but allow some of the substrate to be excreted. We can then write:

$$-\dot{n}_{s,in} \cdot \Delta h_s + \dot{n}_{s,out} \cdot \Delta h_s = \dot{q} + \dot{w}. \quad (5)$$

If we define energy expenditure as in case 1, i.e. as the sum ($\dot{q} + \dot{w}$), it can be seen that it is equivalent to *metabolizeable* energy intake in the stationary isothermal state and, again, that direct and indirect calorimetry measures the same thing. We shall see that this definition of energy expenditure has considerable practical advantages and I will use it in what follows.

Case 3. This case is identical to case 1 except for the fact that we now allow one of the intensive properties of the system to change, namely the average body temperature. We have then:

$$-\overline{C} \cdot d\overline{T}/dt - \dot{n}_{s,in} \cdot \Delta h_s = \dot{q} + \dot{w}. \quad (6)$$

By definition, the energy expenditure is ($\dot{q} + \dot{w}$) as given by direct calorimetry. The result of indirect calorimetry is, as before, given by the term $\dot{n}_s \cdot \Delta h_s$, and this is equal to ($\dot{q} + \dot{w} + \overline{C}\, d\overline{T}/dt$). The *heat production* is $\dot{q} + \overline{C} \cdot d\overline{T}/dt$.

Flow of heat *within* the body is generally not considered to be able to generate chemical or physical work (for definition of work see section 2.2.1). It might therefore seem appropriate to consider the quantity $\overline{C} \cdot d\overline{T}/dt$ to be 'lost' and include this term in the definition of energy expenditure. However, because of the possibility of feedback from the body temperature(s) to energy transduction processes (section 2.2.4), the definition of energy expenditure suggested here is more general.

The different results obtained by direct and indirect calorimetry in this case is not without practical consequences. When measurements are performed over long periods, say 24 h, the difference will in general be negligible: the term $\overline{C} \cdot d\overline{T}/dt$ will be very small compared to the other terms. However, over shorter periods and in connection with physical work the difference may not be small. The problem has been discussed in more detail in a paper by Garby et al. [20] in relation to energy expenditure during sleep.

Case 4. This case is identical to case 1 except that we allow the amount of substrate in the body to change as a result of passive accumulation and deaccumulation by way of combustion. We have

$$dN_s \cdot \Delta h_s/dt - \dot{n}_{s,in} \cdot \Delta h_s = \dot{q} + \dot{w}. \quad (7)$$

In this case, the energy expenditure is given, as before, by the sum ($\dot{q} + \dot{w}$) and equally observed by direct and indirect calorimetry.

Case 5. In this case, we admit the possibility of accumulation of energy in products due to formation from reactants, e.g. protein molecules from amino acids. This requires extra terms on the left side of the equation, i.e. terms of the form $dN \cdot \Delta h_r/dt$, where Δh_r is the energy of formation of the product, N, from its reactants. The energy necessary for these reactions is taken from other reactions where substrate undergoes combustion. The energy expenditure, i.e. the sum ($\dot{q} + \dot{w}$), is not obtained by indirect calorimetry. As an example, consider the (theoretical) situation where all the energy of the combusion reaction is 'trapped' in, e.g., adenosine triphosphate (ATP). In this case, the sum ($\dot{q} + \dot{w}$) is zero but the term $\dot{n}_{s,in} \cdot \Delta h_s$, which is the quantity observed by indirect calorimetry, is not. The energy transformations following a meal show this phenomenon [24b].

This case can be further developed in terms of formation, with or without subsequent excretion, of any compounds. An important special case is that of excretion of breast milk. Here, the energy lost is taken to be equal to the heat of combustion times a factor of 1.25 to account for the extra costs of synthesis. It should be noted that the energy expenditure in this case is not given by the sum ($\dot{q} + \dot{w}$), but as the sum ($\dot{q} + \dot{w} - 1.25 \cdot \Sigma \dot{n}_{s,out} \cdot \Delta h_s$).

Case 5 illustrates a situation where measurements of energy expenditure by means of indirect calorimetry cannot, in general, be expected to measure the same quantity as the sum ($\dot{q} + \dot{w}$). It is, however, important to note that, in the case of normal subjects observed over a period of 2–3 days, it has been shown [1, 4] that the time-averaged net energy supply, i.e. the sum of the three terms $-\Sigma \dot{n}_{net} \cdot \Delta h - \dot{q} - \dot{w}$ (where the summation is over all three substrates), was found to be equal to the time-averaged net energy accumulation, $-\Sigma \Delta h \; dN/dt$ (where again the summation is over all the three substrates). The experiments were performed over periods of net energy deaccumulation of up to 10 MJ/day and with net energy accumulation of up to 2 MJ/day. These results clearly show that, under the conditions mentioned, the net energy transformations in humans can be described completely in terms of the main three substrate, i.e. carbohydrates, fats and proteins. In agreement with the above data, Dauncey [10a] showed that direct and indirect calorimetry provided identical results in normal subjects in approximately zero energy balance when the measurements were averaged over 24 h.

There are no systematic data concerning the relationship between direct and indirect calorimetry over shorter periods of study. Interpretation of such studies are extremely difficult because of the uncertainty with which the term $\overline{C} \cdot d\overline{T}/dt$ can be observed over shorter intervals (hours).

This section can now be summarized as follows: the term energy expenditure can be defined operationally and is in many, but not all, situations obtained equally by direct and by indirect calorimetry.

2.2. Relation between Energy Expenditure and Efficiency of Energy Transduction

The energy expenditure is a direct measure of the cost of running the body machinery including performance of external work. It is also a measure of the rate at which the body must receive metabolizeable energy from food in order to maintain the situation – whatever the situation may be.

The concept of metabolic adaptation implies that the costs may be different among subjects because of differences in the previous history of energy intake with the implication that the efficiency of energy utilization is different. This section deals with the concept of energy utilization or, better expressed, energy transduction.

The First Law, as expressed in section 2.1 (equation 2) for the human body, states that when the body transforms chemical energy in the food (or in the body) into heat and into external work, the total energy is conserved. The First Law has, however, nothing to say about the relative magnitudes of these latter two forms of energy. Also, it has nothing to say about *how* this transformation occurs and, most importantly, about the *results of the transformations with respect to the chemical, physico-chemical and physical state of the body.* In this sense, the First Law, although being an important book-keeping device, is of little direct relevance to problems of energy transformation.

The chemical, physico-chemical and physical state of the body is essentially unstable: the structures are made up of generalized potentials that are far from equilibrium and thus have a tendency to breakdown. The structures are, however, maintained because they are coupled to reactions which continuously receive reactants by external supply of substrate (= energy). In addition to this most important result, three other results are obvious: (1) maintenance of a body temperature which, in general, is different from the surroundings; (2) performance of external work; (3) production and release of specific chemical components, e.g. milk. The last three results are straightforward, but the first needs clarification.

2.2.1. Stationary Non-Equilibria and Work Potentials

Consider a closed system of water to which we add the chemical compound AB. This compound will react to form the products A and B:

$$AB \rightleftharpoons A + B, \tag{8}$$

and the process will continue until the reaction comes to equilibrium. At this point, the relation between the concentrations (or, more rigorously, the activities) c_{AB}, c_A and c_B becomes constant and we can write:

$$\frac{c_A^{eq} \cdot c_B^{eq}}{c_{AB}^{eq}} = k, \tag{9}$$

where k is the equilibrium constant of the reaction and the superscripts indicate that the concentrations are those at equilibrium.

Before the reaction comes to equilibrium, i.e. at any time the product of the concentrations c_A and C_B is smaller than the expression $k \cdot c_{AB}$, the reaction proceeds spontaneously towards the right. Conversely, if we have started the reaction by adding the species A and B to the water, the reaction would proceed towards the left. In the latter case, also, the reaction would be spontaneous.

The preceding paragraph leads up to one of the most important statements of thermodynamics, namely that *any spontaneous reaction can, in principle, be made to perform work.* This is one of the many equivalent forms of the Second Law of Thermodynamics.

Consider now the previously mentioned system in a situation where the concentrations of AB, A and B at a certain time, t, are such that

$$c_A^a \cdot c_B^a / c_{AB}^a \text{ is less than } k,$$

where the superscripts indicate *actual* concentrations rather than equilibrium concentrations. In this situation there exists, by virtue of the Second Law, *a potential to perform work.* In order to express this potential in a quantitative manner, we consider the expression $c_A^a \cdot c_B^a / c_{AB}^a$ in relation to the expression $c_A^{eq} \cdot c_B^{eq} / c_{AB}^{eq}$ and write for the potential:

$$\Delta G = RT\ln(c_A^a c_B^a / c_{AB}^a) - RT\ln(c_A^{eq} c_B^{eq} / c_{AB}^{eq}).$$

This expression is equal to the amount of work that *can* be obtained from the reaction when one unit of AB, e.g. 1 mol, reacts to form the products A and B. The expression is identical to the well-known thermodynamic potential of Gibbs and the work that *can* be extracted is called *free energy;* in this case it is the free energy of the reaction $AB \rightarrow A + B$.

If, in an open system, it is observed that the *stationary* concentrations of a reaction are such that a potential for work exists, i.e. $\Delta G < 0$, and is maintained, we can conclude that energy, e.g. in the form of reactants, is continuously added to the system and that work *can* continuously be extracted from the system.

The above considerations for a simple chemical reaction is equally valid for any process. For example, the condition for transport equilibrium for species distributed across a cell membrane is that the concentrations (or, more rigorously, the activities) on both sides obey the relation:

$$RT \ln c^{I}/c^{II} - zF \cdot \Delta V = 0,$$

where the Roman superscripts refer to the two solutions separated by the membrane, z is the electrical charge of the species, F is the Faraday constant and ΔV is the electrical potential difference between the two solutions. In living systems, it is often observed that this relation is not fulfilled. For example, sodium ions are distributed very unequally between extra- and intracellular fluid. This stationary non-equilibrium state can only exist because energy is continuously being supplied to the system to transport sodium ions out of the cells; work is performed. By the same token, there exists a steady potential for obtaining work by the process with which the sodium ions leak back spontaneously into the cells.

2.2.2. Coupled Processes: Stationary Structures

The fact that a spontaneous process can, in principle, be used to perform work does not imply that work is, in fact, obtained. Work can only be extracted from a spontaneously process if the latter is *coupled* to another process on which the work is made. For example, the reaction between glucose and oxygen in the human body is coupled to another reaction in which adenosine-diphosphate (ADP) is phosphorylated to ATP. In this process, which takes place in the mitochondria of the cells, some of the chemical energy released during combustion is trapped in chemical energy in ATP; the reaction between glucose and oxygen can be said to perform continuous work on the ADP + P $\rightarrow$ ATP system.

The stationary transcellular non-equilibrium of sodium ions is maintained because transport of sodium out of the cells is accomplished by coupling to hydrolysis of ATP and there is thus coupling between the ATP $\rightarrow$ ADP + P system and the Na^+in $\rightarrow$ Na^+out system. We can write:

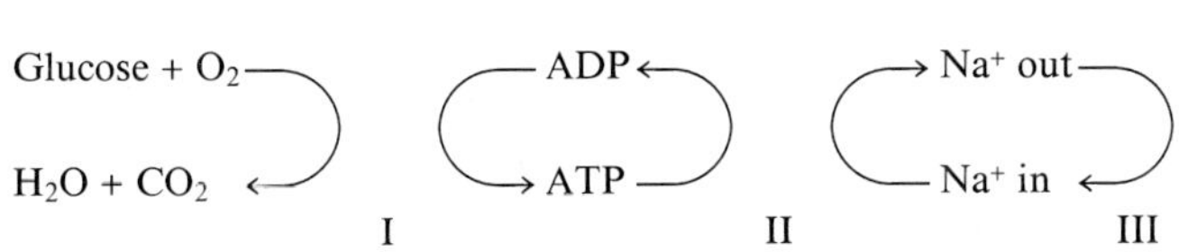

In the above system, we can recognize three steps. There is coupling in steps I and II, whereas there is no coupling in step III; the sodium ions leak back into the cells without performing any work. If we uncouple in step I and let the system go to equilibrium, the total energy of the reaction of glucose + $O_2 \rightarrow H_2O + CO_2$ will be transformed into heat. In the stationary situation with coupling at step I and step II, there will be heat release at both sites, $\dot{q}_I$, and $\dot{q}_{II}$, because coupling can never be complete, i.e. 100% effective. However, the total heat produced by the system will be the sum of the heat evolved in each of the three steps and $-\dot{n}_s \cdot \Delta h = \dot{q}_I + \dot{q}_{II} + \dot{q}_{III}$. The result of the combustion process is the release of heat, at a rate exactly equal to that released were the combustion reaction uncoupled, but we have obtained a system in which there is 'structure', i.e. stationary non-equilibria, both with respect to the ATP $\rightleftarrows$ ADP + P system and the Na^+out $\rightleftarrows$ Na^+in system. Stationary structures of this kind are often called dissipative structures; they disappear when the energy supply ceases.

2.2.3. The Functional Organization of the Energy Transductions in the Body

In this section, I develop the concepts in 2.2.1 and 2.2.2 and describe the most important elements of energy transduction in the body and the functional relationship between these elements. The total heat output is shown to be a sum of heat produced at several levels. The description forms the basis for an analysis of the possible structure of *the control system* in 2.2.4 and, therefore, of the possible sites of metabolic adaptation. A schematic diagram of the salient features of the system is shown in figure 1.

Step 1. Substrate molecules (carbohydrate, fat and protein) and oxygen enter the body and react to produce products that are eliminated. This reaction is spontaneous with a value of ΔG which is very nearly identical to the value of the energy (enthalpy) of the reaction, Δh. Work is produced because the reaction is coupled to the reaction where ADP is phosphorylated to ATP. The coupling is fairly inefficient and some of the energy released in the combustion reaction appears as heat, $\dot{q}_1$.

Step 2. Next, the ATP molecules are hydrolysed to produce ADP and P. This reaction is spontaneous under the conditions that exist in vivo and is thus able to produce work. This work is performed by coupling of the reaction to a large number of different reactions (or processes) of which only the most important are shown in the figure 1.

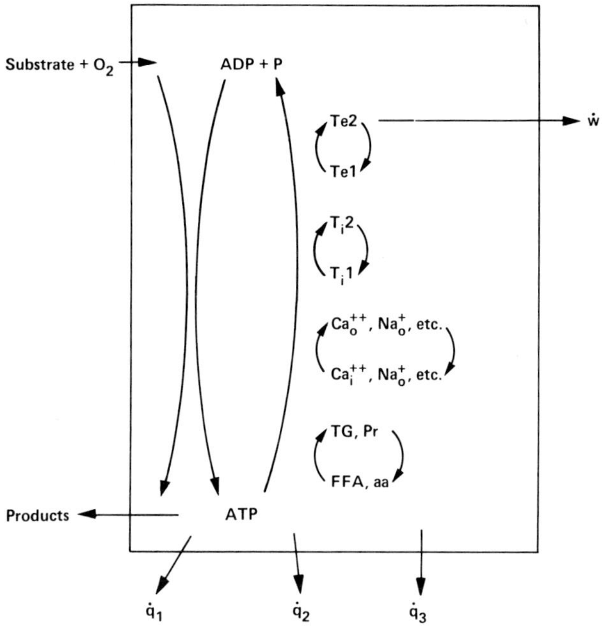

Fig. 1. A schematic diagram of the functional organization of the most important energy transductions in the body. Substrate and oxygen enter the system and react to form products that are excreted. The reaction is spontaneous and is coupled to the formation of ATP from ADP + P. Hydrolysis of ATP is spontaneous and coupled to a number of processes. The process tel → Te2 represents contraction of skeletal muscles with further mechano-mechanical coupling to external work, $\dot{w}$. Relaxation of this process is spontaneous. The process $T_i1 \rightarrow T_i2$ represents similar contraction to internal mechanical work and, again, the relaxation is spontaneous. The process $Ca_i^{2+} \rightarrow Ca_o^{2+}$ represents translocation of Ca^{2+} ions (and other ions) against an electrochemical gradient. The reverse process is spontaneous. The process FFA → TG (and amino acids to protein) represents synthesis and the reverse process is spontaneous.

The first of these processes consists of transduction of the chemical energy in the ATP → ADP + P system to mechanical work in muscles and subsequent mechano-mechanical coupling to external work. The potential here is a time-averaged value of the tension in relation to that at rest. Neither coupling is perfect and there is a heat production, $\dot{q}_2'$.

The second of these processes is similar to that of the first, except that no external work is performed. The heat produced is $\dot{q}_2''$.

The third process consists of transduction of the chemical energy in the ATP → ADP + P system to the transport of several ions, e.g. Na^+, K^+ and Ca^{2+}. The stationary distribution of these ions across membranes is far from equilibrium. Pumping of ions is not perfect and heat $\dot{q}_2'''$ is released.

The fourth process consists of synthesis of chemcial compounds, e.g. triglycerides (TG) from fatty acids (FFA) and glycerol and proteins (Pr) from amino acids, respectively. Heat $\dot{q}_2''''$ is released in these synthetic processes.

Step 3. In this step, the processes in step 2 are relaxed such that the potentials achieve stationary values; transported ions leak back and molecules synthesized in step 2 are broken down. These processes are spontaneous and uncoupled and heat $\dot{q}_3 = \dot{q}_3' + \dot{q}_3'' + ...$ is released.

Although the energy transduction processes shown in the figure presumably represent the quantitatively most important in the overall transduction, two other processes should be mentioned. Complete uncoupling in step 1 takes place in brown adipose tissue. Hydrolysis of ATP without further coupling also takes place in the so-called futile cycles. The relative importance of these two phenomena remains unsettled, but the first is presumably negligible in adult humans.

A most important potential, i.e. the thermal potential or the average body temperature, remains to be mentioned. Clearly, the heat generated during the energy transductions can be used to maintain a body temperature that is above that of the surroundings.

A fundamental property of the system depicted in figure 1, namely the relative magnitudes of the flow of energy and heat in each of the different processes, is known to a very limited extent only. The amount of energy used for external work is small in most individuals of most Western societies, of the order of a few percent of the resting metabolic rate. The amount of internal mechanical work is also small, of the order of 10–15% of the energy expenditure at rest, and is mainly concerned with the maintenance of muscular tonus and with the propulsion of blood, intestinal content and urine. The work associated with translocation of Na^+ ions appears to be very small indeed, of the order of 5–10% of the total energy consumed at rest. However, the work performed in translocation of Ca^{2+} ions may be larger [8]. The work performed on the triglyceride/fatty acid cycle is presumably very small, of the order of 0.5% of the total energy expenditure at rest [13]. The work performed on the amino acid/protein cycle has been calculated to be of the order of 10–15% of the total energy expenditure [41], but there are suggestions that this number may be too small [34, 43].

At the present time, we have to admit a rather profound ignorance about the relative magnitude of the different processes that transform energy. Perhaps the most likely candidates for a major contribution are (1) turnover of the amino acid/protein cycle, and (2) translocation of Ca^{2+} ions across cell membranes.

Girardier [27] has made the interesting point that the heat production of homeothermic animals is about 5 times higher than that of a poikilothermic animal of the same size and temperature. He has also suggested that this may indicate that normal metabolism of homeothermic animals is under *continuous stimulation* in order to maintain the body temperature. In view of the discussion above, one might speculate that protein turnover or Ca^{2+} ion translocation are the stimulated processes.

2.2.4. Regulation and Control of the Energy Potentials

It is very plausible to assume that a large number of the energy potentials mentioned in the previous section requires mechanisms to ensure that they are kept at constant, or nearly constant, values despite perturbations in energy supply or energy expenditure. Part of a few of the mechanisms involved here has been studied, e.g. control of the energy intake by the so-called appetite and control of the heat loss by skin blood flow and sweating, but it is fair to say that present knowledge is far from satisfactory. *It is a fundamental feature of the concept of metabolic adaptation that important mechanisms in the regulation of energy potentials consist of control of the efficiency of the energy transductions* and a discussion of the control system is therefore mandatory.

Intensive properties such as temperature, pressure and Gibbs potentials can be kept at reasonably constant values in spite of perturbations in the flow of energy when they are associated with large capacity factors, i.e. heat capacity, volume and amount of matter, respectively. In this way, relatively large amounts of energy in the form of heat or chemical energy can be accumulated, or deaccumulated, without large changes in the corresponding potentials. This is true for the thermal potential and the potentials associated with fat and glycogen. The corresponding capacity elements in the body (= stores) are presumably very important mechanisms for 'protecting' the more critical potentials, e.g. those associated with the non-equilibria of Na^{+}, K^{+} and Ca^{2+}. However, if, as generally assumed, these elements function as passive buffers, the end result cannot be classified as *regulation* in the general language of control theory. Here, regulation implies maintenance of a particular intensive property by (1) detection, (2) feedback, (3) integration and (4) control by means of effector mechanisms.

As mentioned above, any potential that requires regulation needs to be measured and the information needs to be fed back to some centre for comparison and integration with subsequent transmission of signals to effector organs. At the present time, the control system must be assumed to operate according to the schematic diagram of figure 2. Inclusion in this diagram of control by way of variability of the coupling in the processes B → A and A → B is not a requirement for independent regulation of T_i and A/B. However, this possibility must be considered because it provides the system with increased freedom and it is in keeping with the growing realization that control systems in the body in general are redundant.

Payne and Dugdale [37] have described a model for energy metabolism containing elements which can account for differences in energy expenditure between subjects due to differences in the use of specified metabolic pathways. The authors correctly point out that the commonly used notion of zero energy balance, i.e. stationary conditions with respect to total energy content, is entirely compatible with cyclic changes in body energy content over shorter time intervals, e.g. 24 h, and that energy may be temporarily accumulated and deaccumulated over a time period with the time integral of body energy content equal to zero. In this situation, the energy expenditure over the time interval will depend on the nature of the compound, i.e. protein or fat, being cycled. The authors were able to show that their model could account for a variety of observed data, in particular the differences between the subjects in the semistarvation study of Keys et al. [29]. The model does not contain any elements of feedback and cannot therefore predict metabolic adaptation in the strict sense. However, provision of a simple feedback loop to the process governing the relative magnitude of the two pathways makes the model complete in this sense and provides an additional mechanism for metabolic adaptation.

The control system depicted in figure 2 may now be viewed in relation to the idea of Girardier [27] (section 2.2.3). If the problem of keeping a body temperature constant, and generally higher than that of the environment, was 'solved' by evolution through inefficient coupling, it is highly unlikely that coupling efficiency became fixed. Furthermore, the question of 'why we eat?' takes an interesting direction. Do we eat mainly because

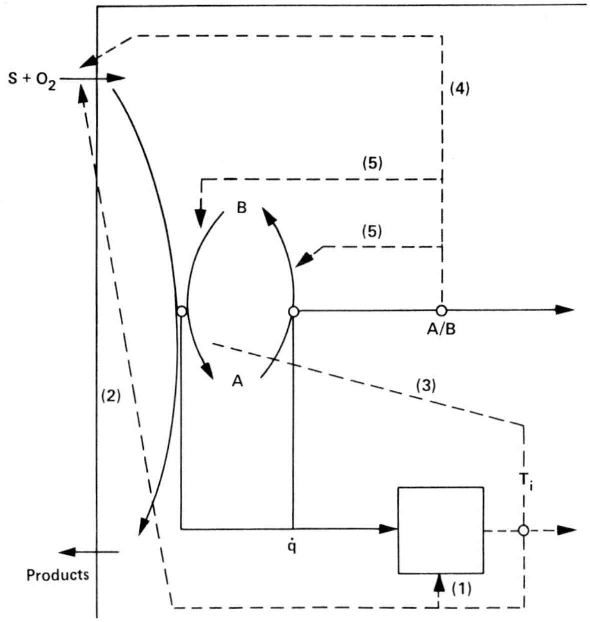

Fig. 2. A schematic diagram of the principles of regulation and control of the energy exchange and transformations in the human body. The diagram illustrates the main features of the system shown in figure 1, but the thermal potentials, is included explicitly and, for simplicity, only one of the other potentials A/B, is included. The system regulates both T_i and A/B. Information about T_i is fed to (1) the skin (blood flow and evaporation); (2) the food energy intake, and (3) the efficiency of maintaining the potential A/B. Information about A/B is fed to (4) the energy intake and (5) the efficiency of maintaining A/B. Regulation of T_i and A/B is independent despite the fact of the common elements.

we need to produce so much heat and do we, in consequence thereof, get the energy potentials without extra costs? Are we constantly trying to uncouple in order to prevent the energy potentials from becoming too large?

The fundamental feature of the concept of metabolic adaptation is that control of the efficiency of the energy transductions is a very important mechanism of regulation of the energy potentials. If the degree of coupling is controlled by feedback, the relation between energy supply and the magnitude of the regulated energy potentials may become *highly non-*

linear and potentials may be maintained at near-constant values despite large fluctuations in energy supply (or energy expenditure). If this is the case, it follows that a steady perturbation can induce a new stationary state with practically identical critical potentials. This is adaptation without costs.

3. Operational Definitions of Metabolic Adaptation

The concept of metabolic adaptation developed in the preceding sections can now be stated as follows. The human body can adapt to changes in energy intake through mechanisms that change the efficiency of the energy transductions in such a way that the energy potentials are maintained.

It is not possible at the present time to provide direct experimental evidence for the existence of such mechanisms in relation to defined steps of energy transduction. In this sense, the definition above is conceptual rather than operational.

It is, however, possible to define the concept in operational terms if we are willing to substitute the notion of maintained energy potentials by the notion of maintained *performance* and if we believe that performance can be defined in physiologically meaningful terms. Any performance of the body can then be regarded as an *output* and it can be related to its *costs,* i.e. its energy expenditure. The concept of metabolic adaptation is then identical to the sentence above with the words *energy potentials* substituted by the word *performances.*

A number of activities of the human body can be defined such that they fulfil both the requirement of being of practical interest and of being reproducible. These activities include rest, a number of defined single activities involving physical work and, finally, a combination of such activities into a fixed programme over a time interval, e.g. 24 h.

The phenomenon of metabolic adaptation can therefore be said to have occurred whenever the energy expenditure of a given performance has changed (or is different) as a result of a change (or a difference) in energy intake. The extent of metabolic adaptation is given directly by the observed change (or difference) in energy expenditure, e.g. as a percentage.

The definition of metabolic adaptation used here, i.e. maintained performance at lower costs, is complete in the sense that it can be observed and that it has a well-understood physiological meaning. However, a word of caution is needed. Definition of adaptation and adapted states in terms of control theory do not imply that the system as such is maintained: the general relation between perturbations and responses must be assumed to depend on the capacity of the effector mechanisms and this cannot be assumed to be infinitely large. Thus, any adapted state will, in principle, have a lower capacity to respond to a new perturbation (in the same direction) and, in this sense, adaptation cannot be assumed to be without costs.

The energy expenditure of a given subject depends on a number of factors not related to the previous history of energy intake. It is clear, therefore, that the effects of these other factors must be eliminated, either by experimental design or by appropriate correction factors. This is discussed below.

3.1. Determinants of Energy Expenditure

Aside from the hypothetical dependency of the energy expenditure on the previous history of food energy intake, the energy expenditure of an individual is known to be related to a number of factors. The most important of these are (1) the physical activity; (2) the body mass and composition; (3) the ambient temperature and (4) the recent (hours) food energy intake. Other factors have been invoked, such as (5) sex (6) age and (7) ethnic origin, but it is not clear at the present time whether these factors are related to the energy expenditure directly or indirectly, e.g. by way of the body composition. Each of the factors (1–7) will be discussed below with particular attention to the possibilities of eliminating their effects in studies of the possible importance of metabolic adaptation.

3.1.1. The Relation between Energy Expenditure and Physical Activity

This relation is qualitatively well established and can be understood in a qualitative way. It is almost always the case that physical activity is associated with an increase in the rate of work performed on the surroundings, i.e. the term $\dot{w}$ in the preceding equations. In this way, physical activity will almost always be associated with an increase in the energy expenditure through this term. It should, however, be pointed out that the relation between the term physical activity and the term external work is not simple. Maintenance of the body, or part thereof, in a fixed position is certainly associated with physical work and an increase in energy expenditure, but no external work is performed and $\dot{w} = 0$. The internal mechanical work in such a situation is dissipated as heat within the body and this heat will appear as an increased rate of heat leaving the body. In fact, by far the largest part of the increase in energy expenditure associated with most forms of physical activity is an increase in the heat produced within, and lost from, the body.

It is difficult to ensure identical physical activity between subjects or within one subject at different times, but it is highly likely that a proper design and detailed instructions can make the effect of differences very small. In fact, observations of the *within* subjects variation in energy expenditure over 24 h with fixed physical activity programmes and with measurements performed one week apart show that this variation is very small, about 1–2% (coefficient of variation) [9, 19]. The *between* subjects variation, in subjects with the same body weight and sex, is larger, about 7% (coefficient of variation) [22], but part of this variation is due to measurement error and differences in body composition. The influence of moderate movements during sitting has recently been studied by Kurzer [30]. Her data indicate that instructions to subjects will make the effect of unintentional small movements quite small.

Complicated and not commonly used movements are associated with an energy expenditure that can decrease because of training. This process is, at least partly, interpreted as a result of a more efficient mechano-mechanic coupling and cannot therefore be classified as metabolic adaptation. Such movements or activities should be avoided in studies of metabolic adaptation.

3.1.2. The Relation between Energy Expenditure and Body Mass and Composition

This relationship is only partly understood. The fact that the energy expenditure, for a given physical activity, is larger when the body mass is larger is self-evident, but the relation between the two is not simple. This can be appreciated by considering the following general expression for the energy expenditure (EE) at any given physical activity (or activity programme):

$$EE = \Sigma k_i M_i, \quad (10)$$

where k_i is the energy expenditure, per unit of mass, of the i:th tissue and M_i is the mass of this tissue. The body weight is:

$$M = \Sigma M_i, \quad (11)$$

and the expression of equation 10 can be rewritten as

$$EE = M \cdot 3m \Sigma k_i f_i \qquad (12)$$

where f_i is the fraction of the body weight of the i:th tissue. The derivative of EE with respect to M is:

$$dEE/dM = \Sigma k_i f_i . \qquad (13)$$

The form of equation 13 suggests that the commonly used practice of 'normalizing' an observed energy expenditure by dividing it with the body weight can lead to erroneous conclusions. This statement is further substantiated by the fact that the empirical relations between energy expenditure and body weight, both at rest and at physical work, can be described by the form:

$$EE = aM + b, \quad \text{with} \quad b \neq 0. \qquad (14)$$

Thus, the energy expenditure per unit of body weight is not a constant but varies with body weight and 'normalizing' energy expenditure by division with the body weight is a nonesensical operation.

At the present time, there are no methods available to determine all the fractions f_i in vivo. Methods have, however, been developed to estimate the body composition in terms of two different tissues, fat and fat-free masses. Based upon such measurements and measurements of the energy expenditure at rest and at light physical acitvity programmes over 24 h, the energy expenditure of fat and fat-free tissues have recently been estimated [24a]. At rest, fat tissue was found to have an energy expenditure of 0.31 W/kg and the corresponding value for fat-free tissue was found to be 1.35 W/kg. The associated standard errors of estimate were 0.074 and 0.073 W/kg, respectively. For two different 24-hour fixed programmes of activity with total average energy expenditures of 1.38 × BMR and 1.53 × BMR, the corresponding values were found to be 0.63 and 0.96 W/kg for fat tissue and 1.86 and 2.14 W/kg for lean tissue with standard errors of about 0.5 and 0.90 and 0.12 and 0.13 W/kg, respectively.

It is not possible to ensure identity in body composition between subjects or within subjects at different times. However, whenever these differences are small, the correction factors developed by Garby et al. [24a] will at least partly eliminate the effect. This problem is central to the possibilities of observing the phenomenon of metabolic adaptation and will be discussed in more detail in relation to the actual observations in section 5.

3.1.3. The Relation between Energy Expenditure and Ambient Temperature

This relation has been studied in some detail with respect to acute perturbations in naked subjects. Below and above a zone of 'comfortable' temperature, the energy expenditure is increased. The physiological basis for this phenomenon is at least partly understood. However, because people under real-life conditions adjust their clothing to maintain a 'comfortable microclimate', i.e. the temperature and humidity between the clothing and the skin, the relation between ambient temperature and energy expenditure is not simple. It has not been studied systematically. In any case, measurements of energy expenditure should be performed at controlled ambient temperature and clothing.

There is also a (small) effect on the energy expenditure of ambient humidity [21] and this parameter should also be controlled.

3.1.4. The Relation between Energy Expenditure and Recent Food Intake

Ingestion of a meal is generally associated with an increase in the rate of combustion of substrates, as calculated by indirect calorimetry, and 5–15% of the combustion energy in the meal is transformed within the next 2–5 h. However, only about half of the transformed energy appears as heat during the period [24b] and the increase in energy expenditure is therefore rather small. Nevertheless, the design of experiments to test the hypothesis of metabolic adaptation should take the phenomenon into consideration.

3.1.5. The Relation between Energy Expenditure and Sex and Age

The qualitative aspects of these relations are well documented, but the interpretations are difficult. The relations may well be due to differences in body composition. In fact, the results of Garby et al. [24a] with respect to the differences in energy expenditure between fat and fat-free tissue and the well known differences in body composition between men and women in this respect explain to a very large extent the well-known differences in energy expenditure at rest between men and women. Clearly, experiments to evaluate causes of differences in energy expenditure should be performed on subjects matched with respect to both sex and age.

3.1.6. The Relation between Energy Expenditure and Ethnic Factors

Relatively few studies have been carried out to investigate racial differences in energy expenditure. Resting metabolic rate appears to be lower in Indian subjects [31, 38]. Dieng et al. [106] found lower rates of energy expenditure during standing in West African subjects than in French subjects. Geissler and Aldouri [25] found lower costs of lying, sitting and standing in Asian and African male subjects as compared to European subjects matchend for height, weight and Quetelet index and living in the same climatic conditions. An important observation by McNeill et al. [32] will be discussed in section 5.4.

4. Public Health Significance of the Concept of Metabolic Adaptation

Attempts to estimate the prevalence of energy undernutrition in different communities throughout the world are an important part of the activities of many international and national organizations. Clearly, such data are fundamental to a number of policy decisions.

There are several different ways in which such estimates can be made. In my opinion, a very reasonable approach is that made by the FAO [15]; only this approach will be discussed here and I will summarize the procedure with particular attention to how the concept of metabolic adaptation enters into the problem.

The FAO approach is to define *minimum energy requirements* and then to calculate the prevalence of undernutrition from distribution curves of energy intake. The minimum energy requirements is defined as the energy expenditure of healthy subjects, with no previous history of inadequate energy intake, performing a defined programme of activities over a 24-hour period.

A summary of the activity programme chosen by the FAO to represent minimum maintenance is shown in table 1 [22]. A detailed description of this programme is found in the cited publication.

Since the energy expenditure depends on body weight, body composition, age and sex (section 3.1), the FAO adopted the convention to express energy expenditure as multiples of the resting metabolic rate (BMR or RMR). This procedure entails an assumption which will be discussed below.

The energy expenditure of the programme shown in table 1 was observed by direct calorimetry over 24 h at 24 °C and comfortable clothing and humidity (3–11 g/m^3) to be equal to an average of 1.38 $\times$ BMR in

Table 1. Summary of activity program representing minimum maintenance

Activity	Minutes
Sleeping, resting lying	545
Sitting, with small movements only	815
Washing and dressing, toilet activities	10
Walking and intermittent weight lifting (10 kg)	5
Walking with intermittent knee-bending	55
Standing	10

both male and female subjects [22]. In the FAO report, this number was approximated as 1.4 × BMR.

The average value of 1.4 × BMR was shown to be a result of a near Gaussian distribution of individual values with a standard deviation of 0.1 × BMR [22]. Use of the data to establish a 'cut-off' point for defining minimum energy requirements therefore requires an analysis of the causes of the variation.

On the assumption that the average value represents the average of *fixed* individual values, the cut-off point for definition of undernutrition was taken to be equal to this average value, i.e. 1.4 × BMR. Because of the nature of the distribution, the misclassification would be symmetrical.

On the assumption that the observed average value consists of individual values subject to variation because of different states of metabolic adaptation, the cut-off point was taken as 1.4 × BMR minus twice the standard deviation, i.e. 1.2 × BMR. This operation is equivalent to the assumption that *all* subjects are able to adapt to this level of energy expenditure, or that an average adaptation of 15%, with a normal distribution, can take place.

The two different values for the cut-off point obviously generate different estimates for the prevalence of undernutrition. As an example, for developing market economies in 1979–1981, the two values yielded 23 and 15%, respectively, as the prevalence [15].

4.1. Consequences of Expressing the Energy Expenditure as Multiples of BMR

Normalizing energy expenditure in terms of RMR is a very practical operation. The resting metabolic rate can in most cases be predicted with reasonable accuracy on the basis of the body weight, sex and age according to the tables presented by FAO/WHO/UNU Expert Consultation Report [14]. Its use is, however, limited to the situation where the body weight dependency of energy expenditure is the same for the programme as it is at rest. For programmes with low physical activity, e.g. between 1.00 and 1.70 × BMR, this appears to be true [17]. However, for programmes with a larger energy expenditure, in particular programmes involving lifting of the body, the body weight dependency cannot be expected to be the same as that for rest. In fact, observations with the Harvard step test on Indian subjects show that the ratio of the energy expenditure at work to that at rest is markedly associated with body weight [32].

5. *Experimental Observations*

As long back as 1947, Widdowson [44] observed that in a healthy active population of specified age-sex group and engaged in similar work, there are two individuals in every 20, one of whom has a mean weekly intake of twice as large as that of the other. This implies a coefficient of variation for mean weekly intake of the some 20%. Part of this variation must be due to variations in body weight, body composition and physical activity. Sukhatme and Margen [40] have analysed the intake data in a group of young army recruits, reported by Edholm et al. [12]. These subjects were engaged in very similar activities of a group nature such as drill, lectures, meals and games. The coefficient of variation of mean weekly intakes was about 13%. Furthermore, the mean square between weeks for intake was found to be significantly larger than the mean square between days within weeks.

These, and other similar, data for variation in intake make it somewhat unlikely that the energy expenditure depends only on such factors as described above, i.e. physical activity, body mass and composition, relation to recent food intake and ambient air conditions. However, the nature of the data do not permit any quantitative estimates of the effect of other factors, e.g. metabolic adaptations.

Sukhatme and Margen [40] have analysed the data of Edholm et al. [12] in terms of the variation over time of the energy balances over one day. They found that the energy balances over successive days were autocorrelated, i.e. the value on one day depended on the value of the previous day. This finding must be taken as strong evidence that energy balance or, rather, something associated with energy balance, is regulated and it is therefore in agreement with the general scheme of how control is exercised in the system (fig. 2). The phenomenon does not, however, distinguish between the different possibilities of feedback and cannot, therefore, be used as a definite argument for control by way of changes in the energy transductions.

A considerable number of experimental observations have been made on the energy expenditure of different activities, including rest, before and after perturbations of the energy intake. Most of these studies have dealt with observations following a short period of perturbation only and are therefore not easily interpreted in the present context. I have chosen to include only those results with perturbations of more than 20 days.

The observations reviewed below fall into four categories: (1) observations of the energy expenditure before and after a period of excess energy intake; (2) observations of the costs of energy accumulation as a function of energy intake excess with comparison of the results with theoretical calculations of these costs; (3) observations of the energy expenditure before and after a period of decreased food energy intake; (4) observations of the RMR in a group of Indian farmers.

As discussed in detail in section 3, there is a serious problem of interpretation of changes in energy expenditure when there are associated changes in body weight and composition. The problem has no rigorous solution and can be approached only in a semiquantitative way.

5.1. Observations of the Energy Expenditure before and after a Period of Excess Energy Intake

The work of Norgan and Durnin [35]. In this work, 6 young male subjects were observed before and after a period of 42 days of overeating by about 6.2 MJ/day. The average weight increase was 6.03 kg of which 3.7 kg was estimated as fat tissue. The resting metabolic rate increased by an average of 12%. Since the body weight increased by about the same value, the authors concluded that their findings were incompatible with inefficient use of energy. For reasons developed in section 3, this conclusion appears to be erroneous. I have recalculated the data and predicted the increase in the RMR due to changes in body weight and body composition (section 3.1.2). The predicted increase in BMR is 5.2% as compared to the observed increase of 12%. The difference, i.e. 7%, can be interpreted as a result of metabolic adaptation if it is assumed that there were no changes in the composition *within* the fat and the lean body compartments.

The authors also observed changes in energy expenditure at sitting and at walking at 4.0 and 5.6 km/h. The relative increases in energy expenditure were 11.9 and 12%. It is not possible to interpret these results in terms of changes in efficiency since there are no data on the relation between energy expenditure at these activities and body weight and body composition. Any component of metabolic adaptation in these activities must however be smaller than the quoted values.

The work of Welle et al. [42]. In this work, five healthy subjects, three males and two females, overate for 20 days by approximately a 50% increase in their customary energy intake. The fasting metabolic rate increased from an average of 80.2 W to an average of 85.7 W. The average weight increase was 3.1 kg. Prediction of the average resting metabolic rate on the assumption that the weight increase was equally divided between lean and fat tissue [16] gives a value of 82.8 W and a calculated increase due to metabolic adaptation of about 4%. This number would be 5–6% if the weight increase were due to a larger proportion of fat tissue.

The work of Forbes et al. [16]. This paper presents results from their own data as well as from a critical examination of literature data. In their own studies, 13 female and 2 male subjects were overfed by 4–8 MJ/day over a period of 20 days. All subjects increased their weight and the range was 3.5–5.8 kg of which 51% was lean tissue as measured by total body potassium. Using these data and comparable data from the literature (when all of the subjects were considered, lean weight accounted for 38% of the total weight gain), linear regressions of the increase in body weight on excess energy intake were calculated. The costs of weight gain and lean tissue gain were calculated from the slopes of the two regressions. The results were found to be practically identical to theoretical estimates of the costs.

The slopes of the two regression lines are associated with fairly large standard errors of estimates, as judged visually. There is also a problem with respect to the statistical model used for calculating the relation between the two variables and thus the slopes. However, the results clearly do not support the idea that excessive energy intake results in an inefficient use of energy.

The values of the RMR before and after the period of overeating show an increase of 0.49 MJ/day, or 8.7%. The increase can be predicted on the basis of the values referred to in section 3, i.e. 0.118 MJ/day/kg of lean tissue and 0.026 MJ/day/kg of fat tissue. I have made these calculations and have found an increase of 0.32 MJ/day, or 5.7%. The difference between this value and the observed value, i.e. 8.7%, was not statistically significant. On the assumption that the composition of both lean and fat tissue remained the same, the difference of 3% could be assigned to metabolic adaptation. This effect would not be detected in the above described analysis of the cost of deposition.

5.2. Observations of the Costs of Energy Accumulation as a Function of Energy Intake Excess with Comparison of the Result with Theoretical Calculations of These Costs

This work has been described above.

5.3. Observations of the Energy Expenditure before and after a Period of Decreased Food Energy Intake

The work of Benedict et al. [5] deals with results of measurements of the energy expenditure before and after a period with a low energy intake and with considerable weight loss. The measurements were performed on 24 apparently healthy young subjects divided into two groups, A and B. Group A subjects had an initial body weight of 67.0 kg and a habitual food energy intake of 1,847 kcal/day over a period of 120 days and lost an average of 7.2 kg. Group B subjects had an initial average body weight of 67.9 kg and were assumed to have the same habitual food energy intake as group A subjects. They were put on a food energy intake of 1,375 kcal/day over a period of 20 days and lost an average of 4.6 kg. The results in table 2 show a considerable decrease in the energy expenditure. The data in table 3 show that the reduction in BMR is far greater than can be accounted for by usual correction. On this basis, the metabolic adaptation is about 17%.

The work of Beattie and Herbert [3] and of Keys et al. [29]. Pacey and Payne [36] have performed similar calculations on the semistarvation data of Beattie and Herbert [3] and of Keys et al. [29]. They arrived at a figure of 14 and 19% decrease in BMR per unit of body weight, respectively. These estimates are likely to be understimates because of the fact that the relation between BMR and body weight, in the interval considered, has a positive intercept (section 3.1.2). James and Shetty [28] have calculated the decrease in BMR per kg of 'active tissue' (body weight minus sum of fat, bone mineral and extracellular fluid derived by a formula from measurements of total body water and extracellular fluid volume) in the experiments of Keys et al. [29] and arrived at an estimate of 14%, most of which was achieved during the first weeks of the study.

Table 2. Different measurements of the energy expenditure (watts) before and after a period of reduced food energy intake

		1	2	3	4	5
Initial	A	80.8	85.5			85.5
	B			92.2	290	83.5
Final	A	65.6	63.8	74.2	221	66.6
	B			72.2	246	66.8

Column numbers: (1) standard BMA; (2) standard BMR in groups of 12 subjects; (3) standing; (4) walking on treadmill; (5) sleeping in groups of 12 subjects.

Table 3. Average initial and final energy expenditure (watts) and three different ways to predict final energy expenditure

Group A	Initial	83.9			
	Final	65.3	78.6[1]	81.7[2]	74.3[3]
Group B	Initial	83.5			
	Final	66.8	80.1[1]	82.1[2]	77.3[3]

The observed values for group A subjects are the means of columns 1, 2 and 5 in table 2. The observed values for group B are the values of column 5 in table 2.

[1] Predicted on the basis of the regression lines for BMR vs body weight according to the table 5 in FAO/WHO/UNU Expert Consultation [14].

[2] Predicted on the assumption that the weight loss consists of fat only and using a value of 0.31 W/kg fat tissue.

[3] Predicted on the assumption that the weight loss consists of lean tissue only and using a value of 1.35 W/kg of lean tissue.

The work of de Boer et al. [7]. In this work, the 24-hour energy expenditure on a fixed programme was observed in 12 obese women and after a period of 8 weeks weight reduction. The average body weight was initially 93.3 kg with a body fat of 43.8% and after weight reduction 82.5 kg with a body fat of 39.2%. Thus during the weight reduction period, these women lost on an average 2.2 kg lean tissue and 8.6 fat tissue. The energy expenditure decreased from a mean value of 10.52 to 8.92 MJ/day. The data were analysed by comparing the observed energy expenditure after weight reduction to that predicted on the basis of the body composition changes. The prediction was based on a multiple regression of energy expenditure on body weight and body fat obtained from a previous study of 47 lean and overweight women in the same laboratory. The ratio of observed to predicted energy expenditure before weight reduction was 0.987 ± 0.013 (mean and SEM) but decreased to 0.943 ± 0.016 after weight reduction. Thus, the energy expenditure had declined more than could be explained by the change in body weight and body composition. Assuming that there were no changes in the composition within the fat and fat-free tissues, this result is evidence of metabolic adaptation with a magnitude of about 4%.

The work of Doré et al. [11]. In this work, the energy expenditure at rest was observed in 19 obese female subjects before and after a period of about one year of decreased energy intake. The subjects had an initial body weight of 104.5 kg (SD = 9.1 kg) and the average weight loss was 30.8 kg with a range of 10.0–53.4 kg. The average energy expenditure before and after the period of weight reduction was 290 (SD = 33) ml O_2/min, respectively, and every subject showed a decrease. I have predicted the decrease in the energy expenditure on the basis of the observed decreases in fat and fat-free mass and the values referred to above (section 3.1.2). The observed energy expenditure was 1.0 ± 2.0% (mean and standard error of the mean) lower than that predicted.

The work of Garby et al. [23]. The effect of 12 weeks light-moderate underfeeding on the 24-hour energy expenditure of a fixed physical activity programme was studied in 6 male and 6 female subjects. During a control period of 2 weeks, measurements were made of 24-hour energy expenditure by direct calorimetry, the lean and fat body masses and the subjects' habitual energy intakes. The average body weight, expressed as percent of ideal, was 107%, and did not change significantly during the control period. The subjects were asked to continue to record their daily food intake while reducing it by 25% and to continue their daily habits during a period of 12 weeks. The mean change in body weight was −2.9 kg (range from +1.9 to −9.2 kg) with an average change in body energy content of −66 MJ (range from +75 to −219 MJ). The 24-hour energy expenditure was measured three times during the period, i.e. after 4, 8 and 12 weeks from the start of the decreased energy intake, and found to be practically the same as the control value, i.e. with average differences (SD) of −0.2 (3.9), −0.8 (5.7) and +0.6 (4.2)% from the control value. In the 6 subjects who had the largest loss of body weight, this was found to be

5.0 kg, and the mean differences (SD) in energy expenditure were found to be –1.0 (3.4), 0.0 (5.6) and –0.6 (3.9)%, respectively, from the control value. A significant part of the between-subjects variation in the differences from the control value is due to random measurement error and it was concluded that a loss of body energy content of the magnitude reported here, and due mainly to a reduced food intake, does not result in a significant increase in the efficiency of energy conversion, i.e. metabolic adaptation.

The work of Barrows and Snook [2]. In this work, 15 female obese (126% ideal body weight) subjects were placed on a high-protein, low calorie diet for 4–6 months. They lost an average of 16.6. kg fat mass and 3.3 kg fat-free mass. At the end of the study, the RMR had decreased to a value of 64.6 W from a value of 81.7 W. The decrease in RMR predicted on the basis of the values of section 3.1.2 was only 9.6 W, leaving 7.5 W or 10% as metabolic adaptation.

The work of Bessard et al. [6]. In this work, 5 obese women (152% ideal weight) were placed on a low calorie diet for 11 weeks. The average loss of fat mass was 8.6 kg and of fat-free mass 3.5 kg. The resting energy expenditure decreased from an average of 82.7 W to an average of 68.8 W. The predicted energy expenditure was calculated (section 3.1.2) as 75.3 W, resulting in a metabolic adaptation of 8.6%.

The work of Geissler et al. [26]. The energy expenditure over 24 h for three different physical activity programmes (sedentary, normal and normal + aerobics) were measured in 16 post-obese women and in 16 control subjects. The two groups were matched with respect to age (32.2 vs. 31.5 years), height (165 vs. 166 cm), weight (60.8 vs. 61.8 kg) and percentage of fat (28.5 vs. 26.1%). The energy expenditure (± SE) (kcal/day) of the sedentary programme was 1,273 ± 54 and 1,538 ± 69, respectively, of the normal programme 1,601 ± 69 and 1,882 ± 56, respectively, and of the normal + aerobics 1,823 ± 83 and 2,132 ± 65, respectively. There was thus a consistent and significant difference of about 15% which is not explicable in terms of differences in body composition.

5.4. Observations of the RMR in a Group of Indian Farmers

The work of McNeill et al. [32]. The authors report on measurements of the BMR in rural Indian male subjects. Fifty-eight men aged 20-49 years were studied. The mean body weight was 51.6 (SD = 7.2) kg and the mean body mass index was 19.3 (SD = 2.1) kg/m^2. The mean BMR was 5.40 MJ/day with a standard deviation of 0.69 MJ/day.

The observed values of the BMR were compared to those predicted by the FAO/WHO/UNU Expert Consultation Report [14] and it was found that the observed values were on an average 12.1% (SD = 8.8%) below those predicted. This difference was found to be highly significant ($p < 0.001$ by paired t test). This result is of considerable interest. The coefficient of variation of the mean BMR was 12.8% and, with a coefficient of variation of 14% of the body weight, suggests that the variation between subjects of the same body weight must be small indeed. The average difference between the observed and predicted value is quite high and a considerable proportion of the subjects must have had values between 15 and 20% lower than predicted. A mean body mass index of 19.3 kg/m^2 with a mean body weight of 51.6 kg does not suggest that the subjects had more fat tissue than normal.

Table 4. Summary of experimental data

Source	Perturbation	Subjects	Average change in body weight ΔBW (ΔFM + ΔFFM), kg	Difference between observed and predicted energy expenditure[1], %
Norgan and Durnin [35]	overreating	6 M	+6.0 (2.3 + 3.7)	+7
Welle et al. [42]	overeating	3 M + 2 F	+3.1	+5
Forbes et al. [16]	overeating	2 M + 13 F	+4.5 (2.3 + 2.2)	+3
Forbes et al. [16]	cost of weight gain and lean tissue gain identical to theoretical values			
Benedict et al. [5]	undereating	12 M	−7.2	−17
Benedict et al. [5]	undereating	12 M	−4.6	−17
Beattie and Herbert [3]		see section		−13 to −19
de Boer et al. [7]	undereating	12 F obese	−10.8 (2.2 + 8.6)	−4
Doré et al. [11]	undereating	19 F obese	−30.8 (8.1 + 22.7)	−1
Garby et al. [23]	undereating	6 M + 6 F	−2.9 (1.9 + 1.0)	0
Garby et al. [23]	undereating	1 M + 5 F	−5.0 (3.6 + 1.4)	0
Barrows and Snook [2]	undereating	15 F obese	−19.9 (3.3 + 16.6)	−10
Bessard et al. [6]	undereating	5 F obese	−16.1 (3.5 + 8.6)	−9
Geissler et al. [26]	undereating	16 F postobese compared to 16 F controls		−15
McNeill et al. [32]		observed RMR in Indian farmers was an average of 12% lower than predicted		

[1] Energy expenditure was observed over 24 h with fixed physical activity programmes in the studies by de Boer et al. [7], Garby et al. [23] and Geissler et al. [26]. In the other studies, energy expenditure was observed at rest under standardized conditions.

There is, however, a possibility that the calculated average difference between the observed and predicted value may be an overestimation. The prediction of the resting RMR on the basis of body weight according to the FAO/WHO/UNU Report [14] is linear equation with a positive intercept, while the true regression is likely to be curved with a decreasing slope with increasing body weight. Thus, prediction of the RMR from body weights at the lower end of the range may overestimate the RMR.

5.5. Summary of Section 5 and Proposal for an Experimental Design

The experimental observations are summarized in table 4. The results do not give a clear-cut answer to the question of the relative importance of the phenomenon of metabolic adaptation. There may be several reasons for this fact. First, it is entirely possible that the response to a perturbation in the food intake varies between individuals due to factors not yet known. If so, mean values of the relatively small samples can be misleading because of the non-random nature of the selection procedures. Secondly, it is entirely possible that the time constant for the process of adaptation can vary between individuals and it may be very long for some subjects. Thirdly, the correction factors for changes in body weight and body composition are not well established; each of the factors for fat tissue and fat-free tissue are 'lumped'. Finally, the clear-cut results of the studies in the Indian farmers may be interpreted as a genetic phenomenon.

6. Comparison of the Experimental Data with the Proposal of the Fifth World Food Survey [15]

It remains to compare the results of the available experimental data with the proposal of the Fifth World Food Survey [15] that a metabolic adaptation of 0.2/1.4 = 15% is a realistic possibility in many populations in developing countries.

Such a comparison requires a more precise description of the situation of the populations that we have in mind. We can assume that the subjects have had a relatively low food energy intake for a long time and that a stationary state has been developed with the result that their body weights are lower than 'ideal' by perhaps 10–20%. This situation is different from the situations achieved in most of the experimental designs described above. The data in table 4 do not permit rejection of the possibility and they cannot be used to support it. They support the idea that metabolic adaptation can occur but they cannot be used in a quantitative way.

7. Summary and Conclusions

(1) The energy content in food is used in the human body for three main purposes. The first is to maintain the dissipative structures. Most of the structures of the body are of this kind, i.e. they represent stationary non-equilibrium states, or (generalized) stationary potentials, and are inherently unstable. The second is to maintain a body temperature independent of and usually higher than that of the surroundings. The third is to provide energy for performance of external work.

The functional structure of the system providing these results consists of a large number of coupled processes (chemical reactions and translocations), in series and in parallel, whose general nature is well understood but whose quantitative extents are mainly unknown. The coupled processes are driven by the spontaneous reaction of the main substrates with oxygen. Energy flows through the system and is converted to heat (and external work) with simultaneous creation of stationary generalized potentials. For each potential there is an associated flow of energy and the relation between the two is an expression of the efficiency with which the potential is maintained.

The processes giving rise to the potentials are likely to be controlled with respect to the efficiency with which the potentials are maintained. The control is partly provided through feedback from the potentials themselves: the potentials are regulated. In this way, the system can respond in a non-linear fashion to perturbations in the energy intake (or energy expenditure): the potentials are maintained at constant, or nearly constant, values.

The concept of metabolic adaptation implies that control of the efficiency by feedback from the potentials is an important element in the overall regulation of the potentials, including that of the body temperature.

(2) The concept of metabolic adaptation can be framed in such a way that it becomes operational. Quantities such as maintained potentials and efficiency can be revealed in terms of their external manifestations: performance of tasks and associated costs (energy expenditure). A change in

efficiency is defined as a change in cost for given tasks. Performances can be defined such that they are both reproducible and of physiological relevance and costs can be measured. There are several complications associated with this approach to operational definition, the most important being the effect on energy expenditure of changes (or differences) in body composition.

(3) The FAO approach to estimation of prevalence of undernutrition is based on measurements of energy expenditure for given tasks. This approach requires knowledge of the extent of metabolic adaptation. Presently available estimates are based on observations in individuals who are unlikely to have had a history of low energy intake and therefore unlikely to exhibit the phenomenon.

(4) Experimental observations concerning the effect of perturbations of the energy intake on energy expenditure and concerning the energy expenditure of presumably low-energy-intake Indian farmers cannot at the present time be interpreted in a rigorous way. They do, however, allow of a tentative conclusion: energy expenditure at rest decreases (increases) following a reduction (increase) in food energy intake and the RMR in Indian farmers is below the values predicted by observations in subjects of presumably higher energy intake. The magnitude of the effect cannot be well established on the basis of present data but is not likely to be negligible, i.e. below 5%.

(5) The proposal by the Fifth World Food Survey [15] that a metabolic adaptation of 15% is a realistic possibility in many populations of the developing countries cannot be rejected or supported by available experimental data.

References

1 Atwater, W.O.; Benedict, F.G.: Metabolism of matter and energy in the human body. US Dept. Agric. Exp. Stn Bull. 136 (US Govt. Printing Office, Washington 1903).

2 Barrows, K.; Snook, J.T.: Effect of a high-protein, very-low-calorie diet on resting metabolism, thyroid hormones, and energy expenditure of obese middle-aged women. Am. J. clin. Nutr. *45:* 391 (1987).

3 Beattie, J.; Herbert, P.H.: Estimation of the metabolic rate in the starvation state: basal metabolism during recovery from severe malnutrition. Br. J. Nutr. *1:* 1985 (1947).

4 Benedict, F.G.; Milner, R.D.: Experiments on the metabolism of matter and energy

in the human body. US Dept. Agric. Exp. Stn Bull. 175 (US Government Printing Office, Washington 1907).
5 Benedict, F.G.; Moles, W.R.; Orth P.; Smith, H.M.: Human vitality and efficiency under prolonged restricted diet (Carnegie Institution of Washington, Washington 1919).
6 Bessard, T.; Schutz, Y.; Jéquier, E.: Energy expenditure and postprandial thermogenesis in obese women before and after weight loss. Am. J. clin. Nutr. *38:* 680 (1983).
7 Boer, J.O. de; Es, A.J.H. van; Roovers, L.A.; Raaij, J.M.A. van; Hautvast, J.G.A.J.: Adaptation of energy metabolism of overweight women to low-energy intake, studied with whole-body calorimeters. Am. J. clin. Nutr. *44:* 585 (1986).
8 Clausen, T.: Personal communication (1987).
9 Dallosso, H.M.; Murgatroyd, P.R.; James, W.P.T.: Feeding frequency and energy balance in adult males. Hum. Nutr. clin. Nutr. *36C:* 25 (1982).
10a Dauncey, M.J.: Metabolic effects of altering the 24 h energy intake in man, using direct and indirect calorimetry. Br. J. Nutr. *43:* 257 (1980).
10b Dieng, K.; Lemonier, D.; Bleiberg, F.; Brun, T.A.: Differences in the rate of energy expenditure of resting activities between European and African men. Nutr. Rep. int. *21:* 183 (1980).
11 Doré, C.; Hesp. R.; Wilkins, D.; Garrow, J.S.: Prediction of energy requirements of obese patients after massive weight loss. Hum. Nutr. clin. Nutr. *36C:* 41 (1982).
12 Edholm, O.G.; Adam, J.M.; Healy, M.J.R.; Wolff, H.S.; Goldsmith, R.; Best, T.W.: Food intake and energy expenditure of army recruits. Br. J. Nutr. *24:* 1091 (1970).
13 Elia, M.; Zed, C.; Neale, G.; Livesey, G.: The energy cost of triglyceride-fatty acid recycling in nonobese subjects after an overnight fast and four days of starvation. Metabolism (in press).
14 FAO/WHO/UNU Expert Consultation: Energy and protein requirements. Tech. Rep. Ser. No. 724 (WHO, Geneva, 1985).
15 The Fifth World Food Survey (FAO, Rome 1985).
16 Forbes, G.B.; Brown, M.R.; Welle, S.L.; Lipinski, B.A.: Deliberate overfeeding in men and women: energy cost and composition of the weight gain. Br. J. Nutr. *56:* 1 (1986).
17 Garby, L.: Relationship between energy expenditure, expressed as the physical activity index, and body weight at low physical activity programmes. Hum. Nutr. clin. Nutr. *39C:* 455 (1985).
18 Garby, L., Larsen, P.S.: Principles and problems of human energy exchange. Am. J. Physiol. *247:* R366 (1984).
19 Garby, L.; Lammert, O.; Nielsen, E.: Within-subjects between-weeks variation in 24-hour energy expenditure for fixed physical activity. Hum. Nutr. clin. Nutr. *38C:* 391 (1984).
20 Garby, L.; Kurzer, M.S.; Lammert, O.; Nielsen, E.: Energy expenditure during sleep in men and women: Evaporative and sensible heat losses. Hum. Nutr. clin. Nutr. *41C:* 225 (1986).
21 Garby, L.; Lammert, O.; Nielsen, E.: 24-h evaporative and sensible heat losses in relation to ambient humidity at 24 °C in clothed human subjects. Acta physiol. scand. *127:* 167 (1986).

22 Garby, L., Lammert, O.; Nielsen, E.: Energy expenditure over 24 hours on low physical activity programmes in human subjects. Hum. Nutr. clin. Nutr. *40C:* 141 (1986).

23 Garby, L.; Kurzer, M.S.; Lammert, O.; Nielsen, E.: Effect of 12 weeks light-moderate underfeeding on 24 hour energy expenditure in normal male and female subjects. Hum. Nutr. clin. Nutr. *42:* 295 (1988).

24a Garby, L.; Garrow, J.; Jørgensen, B.; Lammert, O.; Madsen, K.; Sørensen, P.; Webster, J.: Relation between expenditure and body composition in man. Specific energy expenditure in vivo of fat and fat-free tissue. Hum. Nutr. clin. Nutr. *42:* 301 (1988).

24b Garby, L.: Energy transformations following a meal. Hum. Nutr. clin. Nutr. (in press).

25 Geissler, C.A.; Aldouri, M.S.H.: Racial differences in the energy cost of standardized activities. Ann. Nutr. Metab. *29:* 40 (1985).

26 Geissler, C.A.; Miller, D.S.; Shah, M.: The daily metabolic rate of the post-obese and the lean. Am. J. clin. Nutr. *45:* 914 (1987).

27 Girardier, L.: The regulation of the biological furnace of warm blooded animals. Experientia *33:* 1121 (1977).

28 James, W.P.T.; Shetty, P.S.: Metabolic adaptation and energy requirements in developing countries. Hum. Nutr. clin. Nutr. *36C:* 331 (1982).

29 Keys, A.; Brozek, J.; Henschell, A.; Mickelson, O.; Taylor, H.L.: The biology of human starvation (University of Minnesota Press, Minneapolis 1950).

30 Kurzer, M.: Effect of small movements on the energy expenditure during sitting. Hum. Nutr. clin. Nutr. *41C:* 403 (1987).

31 Mason, E.D.; Jacob, M.; Balakrishnan, V.: Racial group difference in the basal metabolism and body composition in Indian and European women in Bombay. Hum. Biol. *36:* 374 (1964).

32 NcNeill, G.; Rivers, J..W.; Payne, R.R.; Britto, J.J. de; Abel, R.: Basal metabolic rate of Indian men: no evidence of metabolic adaptation to a low plane of nutrition. Hum. Nutr. clin. Nutr. *41C:* 473–483 (1987).

33 Miller, D.S.: Man's demand for energy; in Blaxter, Food chains and human nutrition (Applied Science Publishers, 1979).

34 Muramatsu, T.; Aoyagi, Y.; Okumura, J.; Tasaki, I.: Contributions of whole-body protein synthesis to basal metabolism in layer and broiler chickens. Br. J. Nutr. *57:* 269 (1987).

35 Norgan, N.G.; Durnin, J.V.G.A.: The effect of 6 weeks of overfeeding on the body weight, body composition and energy expenditure of young men. Am. J. clin. Nutr. *33:* 978 (1980).

36 Pacey, A.; Payne, P.: Agricultural development and nutrition (Hutchinson, London 1985).

37 Payne, P.R.; Dugdale, A.E.: A model for the prediction of energy balance and body weight. Ann. hum. Biol. *4:* 525 (1977).

38 Schofield, W.N.; Schofield, C.; James, W.P.T.: Basal metabolic rate – review and prediction, together with an annotated bibliography of source material. Hum. Nutr. clin. Nutr. *39C:* suppl. 1, pp. 5–31 (1985).

39 Sukhatme, P.V.: The world's hunger and future needs in food supplies. J. R. Stat. Soc. A *124:* 463 (1961).

40 Sukhatme, P.V.; Margen, S.: Autoregulatory homeostatic nature of energy balance. Am. J. clin. Nutr. *35:* 355 (1982).

41 Waterlow, J.C.; Garlick, P.J.; Millward, D.J.: Protein turnover in mammalian tissues and in the whole body (North-Holland, Amsterdam 1978).

42 Welle, S.L.; Seaton, T.B.; Campbell, R.G.: Some metabolic effects of overeating in man. Am. J. clin. Nutr. *44:* 718 (1986).

43 Wheatley, D.N.; Inglis, M.S.: Protein turnover during cell growth: a re-examinaion of the problem of linear incorporation kinetics of radioactively labelled amino acids into protein and its relationship to growth characteristics. Cytobios *47:* 187 (1986).

44 Widdowson, E.M.: Nutritional variability. Proc. Nutr. Soc. *21:* 121 (1962).

Lars Garby, MD, PhD, Department of Physiology, University of Odense,
Campusvej 55, DK–5230 Odense M (Denmark)

Subject Index